Acute Stroke Care

A Manual from the University of Texas-Houston Stroke Team

Ken Uchino, M.D.

Jennifer K. Pary, M.D.

James C. Grotta, M.D.

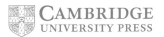

CAMBRIDGE
UNIVERSITY PRESS

CAMBRIDGE UNIVERSITY PRESS
Cambridge, New York, Melbourne, Madrid, Cape Town, Singapore,
São Paulo

Cambridge University Press
The Edinburgh Building, Cambridge CB2 8RU, UK

Published in the United States of America by Cambridge University Press,
New York

www.cambridge.org
Information on this title: www.cambridge.org/9780521674942

First published 2007

Printed in the United Kingdom at the University Press, Cambridge

A catalogue record for this publication is available from the British Library

Library of Congress Cataloguing in Publication data

ISBN 978-0-521-67494-2 paperback

Cambridge University Press has no responsibility for
the persistence or accuracy of URLs for external or
third-party internet websites referred to in this publication,
and does not guarantee that any content on such
websites is, or will remain, accurate or appropriate.

Every effort has been made in preparing this publication to provide accurate
and up-to-date information which is in accord with accepted standards
and practice at the time of publication. Although case histories are drawn
from actual cases, every effort has been made to disguise the identities of the
individuals involved. Nevertheless, the authors, editors and publishers can
make no warranties that the information contained herein is totally free from
error, not least because clinical standards are constantly changing through
research and regulation. The authors, editors and publishers therefore
disclaim all liability for direct or consequential damages resulting from the
use of material contained in this publication. Readers are strongly advised to
pay careful attention to information provided by the manufacturer of any
drugs or equipment that they plan to use.

Acute Stroke Care

You have just encountered a possible stroke patient. You ask yourself, what should I do first? How do I know it is a stroke? Is it too late to reverse the damage? How do I do the right things in the right order? This book will help you answer these critical questions. It provides practical advice on the care of stroke patients in a range of acute settings. As new and effective treatments become available, and designated stroke centers are created, this guidebook will help inform the healthcare professionals responsible for delivering care.

The content is arranged in chronological order, covering the things to consider in assessing and treating the patient in the emergency department, the stroke unit, and then on transfer to a rehabilitation facility. All types of stroke are covered.

A comprehensive set of appendices contain useful reference information including dosing algorithms, conversion factors, and stroke scales.

Ken Uchino is an Assistant Professor of Neurology at the University of Pittsburgh School of Medicine and a Vascular Neurologist at the University of Pittsburgh Medical Center Strohe Institute.

Jennifer Pary is a Vascular Neurologist at the Center for Neurosciences, Orthopedics and Spine, Dakota Dunes, South Dakota.

James Grotta is Professor and Chairman in the Department of Neurology, University of Texas Medical School at Houston.

Cambridge Pocket Clinicians provide practical, portable, note-based guidance for medical trainees, junior doctors, residents, and those from outside the field seeking an accessible overview. Written making maximum use of lists, bullet points, summary boxes and algorithms, they allow the reader fast and ready access to essential information.

Contents

4 TPA protocol   33

5 Neurological deterioration in acute ischemic stroke   48

6 Ischemic stroke prevention: why we do the things we do 61

7 Transient ischemic attack (TIA) 85

8 Intracerebral hemorrhage (ICH) 91

9 Subarachnoid hemorrhage (SAH) 101

10 Organization of stroke care 114

11 Rehabilitation 118

Preface

You have just been called to the emergency department to evaluate and treat a possible stroke patient. You ask yourself: What should I do first? How do I know it is a stroke? Is it too late to reverse the damage, and if not, how do I do it? How do I make sure that I do things correctly during the first day or so to prevent worsening? This handbook is designed to answer these real-life questions. As new and effective stroke treatments are now available, and the creation of designated stroke centers for optimal care of stroke patients is endorsed and put into practice, there is a need for a guidebook that will help enlarge and inform the group of healthcare professionals responsible for delivering this care.

The handbook has been compiled from the day-to-day experiences of the Stroke Team at the University of Texas Medical School – Houston in caring for acute stroke patients on a dedicated in-patient stroke service. It describes the options and underlying rationale for making treatment decisions for stroke patients in the emergency department, stroke unit, neurological critical care unit, and pre-rehabilitation setting. It is evidence-based where evidence exists, but much of what is included reflects our best interpretation of what should be done in the absence of conclusive data.

It is intended as a practical guide to be used by medical students, house officers, and other clinicians with first-hand responsibility for the "nuts and bolts" care of these patients.

The handbook has been arranged generally in chronological order, covering the things one should consider in assessing and treating the patient in the emergency department (ED), then the stroke unit, and then on discharge or transfer to a rehabilitation facility.

Having dealt with the diagnosis of stroke and the essential first steps in the emergency department, we then consider the management of each type of stroke in turn. We begin with ischemic stroke, followed by separate chapters detailing several important issues in ischemic stroke management; the use of thrombolytic therapy, how to approach neurological deterioration, selecting appropriate secondary stroke prevention, and, finally, transient ischemic attack. Then we move on to intracerebral hemorrhage and subarachnoid hemorrhage, before ending chapters on how to organize stroke care and the principles of rehabilitation and stroke recovery.

There is more detail in the ischemic stroke chapter because it represents the initial and most complex decision-making in the ED. When called to the ED to see an acute stroke patient, most often it will be an ischemic stroke, and since the therapy for this condition is most urgent, you should start by assuming it is an ischemic stroke. If, during your evaluation of the patient, you determine that the patient has a TIA or hemorrhage, then many of the same principles outlined in the ischemic stroke chapter also will apply, but you will find specific information for patients with TIA or hemorrhage in their appropriate chapters.

The appendices contain useful reference information that is referred to in the text but is detailed and hard to remember, such as dosing algorithms and conversion factors, standing orders, drug protocols, various stroke scales, and detailed description of imaging sequences and brainstem syndromes.

* In the text, an asterisk marks where there is sufficient evidence to make a strong recommendation based on randomized trials or consensus statements. However, for most decisions, such data do not exist, and we have not hesitated to include our advice based on our collective experiences, and observations of where mistakes are frequently made, and we have emphasized by bold lettering some of those areas where there are particular important values or pieces of information that can help facilitate proper treatment and avoid errors.

We emphasize that this is a **manual for acute stroke diagnosis and treatment**, and hence some disclaimers are needed for what this work does **not** cover. We presume the reader has a basic knowledge of neuroanatomy and vascular physiology, covered in medical and nursing school curricula. None of this is covered, though we provide a refresher for vascular anatomy in an appendix. Similarly, we presume the reader has a basic knowledge of the neurological examination and its common findings in stroke patients, covered in courses on physical diagnosis. Again, this is not covered, though we provide a review of some of the more rare brainstem syndromes in an appendix. Finally, we recognize that a detailed description of the epidemiology, pathology, and outcome of stroke and all of its subtypes, and even many aspects of its diagnosis, treatment, and prevention are left uncovered. For these, we refer the reader to standard excellent texts on cerebrovascular disease.

We hope that this work will help the reader become more comfortable in dealing with the complexities of urgent decision-making, thereby increasing the number of medical personnel engaged in providing acute stroke care, with the end result of reducing the devastation caused by stroke in our society.

Abbreviations

ACA	anterior cerebral artery
ACE	angiotensin converting enzyme
AHA	American Heart Association
ARR	absolute risk reduction
ASA	American Stroke Association
AVM	arteriovenous malformation
CBC	complete blood count
CBV	cerebral blood volume
CEA	carotid endarterectomy
CN	cranial nerve
CPP	cerebral perfusion pressure
CSF	cerebrospinal fluid
CT	computed tomography
CTA	CT angiography
CUS	carotid ultrasound
DBP	diastolic blood pressure
DSA	digital subtraction angiography
DVT	deep venous thrombosis
ED	emergency department
EEG	electroencephalogram
EKG	electrocardiogram
FDA	Food and Drug Administration (USA)
FFP	fresh frozen plasma

GCS	Glasgow coma scale
HIT	heparin-induced thrombocytopenia
HITTS	heparin-induced thrombocytopenia with thrombotic syndrome
IA	intra-arterial
ICA	internal carotid artery
ICH	intracerebral hemorrhage
ICP	intracranial pressure
ICU	intensive care unit
IM	intramuscular
INR	international normalized ratio
IV	intravenous
IVH	intraventricular hemorrhage
LDL	low-density lipoprotein
LMN	lower motor neuron
LTAC	long-term acute care
MAP	mean arterial pressure
MCA	middle cerebral artery
MI	myocardial infarction
MRA	magnetic resonance angiogram
MRI	magnetic resonance imaging
NIH	National Institutes of Health
NIHSS	National Institutes of Health Stroke Scale
NINDS	National Institute of Neurological Disorders and Stroke
NNH	number needed to harm
NNT	number needed to treat
NPO	nil per os (nil by mouth)
OT	occupational therapy
PCA	posterior cerebral artery
PEG	percutaneous endoscopic gastrostomy
PFO	patent foramen ovale

PO	per os (by mouth)
PT	physical therapy
PTT	partial thromboplastin time
RLS	right-to-left shunt
RRR	relative risk reduction
SAH	subarachnoid hemorrhage
SBP	systolic blood pressure
SC	subcutaneous
SNF	skilled nursing facility
ST	speech therapy
TCD	transcranial Doppler ultrasound
TEE	transesophageal echocardiogram
TIA	transient ischemic attack
TPA	tissue plasminogen activator
TTE	transthoracic echocardiogram

Stroke in the emergency department

Stroke is the most common neurological emergency, and, because effective treatment is available that must be started within minutes, most acute neurological presentations should be assumed to be a stroke until proven otherwise by history, exam, or radiographic testing. Unfortunately, there is not a quick and easy laboratory or clinical test to determine for sure that the patient lying in front of you is having a stroke, so an accurate history and exam are essential.

■ Is this a stroke?

DEFINITION

The term "stroke" usually refers either to a cerebral infarction or to non-traumatic cerebral hemorrhage. Depending on the population you are seeing (ethnicity, age, comorbidities) the ratio of infarcts to hemorrhages is about 4:1.

As will be described in more detail in Chapter 3, cerebral infarcts can be caused by a number of pathological processes, but all end with an occlusion of a cerebral artery or vein. If the arterial occlusion results in a reduction of blood flow insufficient to cause death of tissue (infarction), it is termed "ischemia."

As will be described in more detail in Chapter 8, non-traumatic cerebral hemorrhages are caused by a number of pathological processes which all lead to bleeding into the brain parenchyma and ventricles. Bleeding into the subarachnoid space (Chapter 9) is usually caused by a ruptured aneurysm or vascular malformation. Other types of brain bleeding, for example into the subdural or epidural space, are usually traumatic and are not considered in this book.

PRESENTATION

When taking the history, the most characteristic aspect of a cerebral infarct or hemorrhage is the abrupt onset, so be sure to get the exact flavor of the onset. It is also imperative to determine as precisely as possible the time of onset. The symptoms most often stay the same or improve somewhat over the next hours, but may worsen in a smooth or stuttering course. Ischemic strokes (but not hemorrhages) may rapidly resolve, but even if they resolve completely, they may recur after minutes to hours.

The second characteristic historical aspect of cerebral infarcts is that the symptoms will usually fit the distribution of a single vascular territory. This is also the most important characteristic of the neurological exam in a patient with an infarct. Therefore, patients with an infarct will present with symptoms and signs in the middle, anterior, or posterior cerebral arteries, a penetrating artery (producing a "lacunar" syndrome), or the vertebral or basilar artery (see below).

Parenchymal hemorrhages also occur in characteristic locations, and usually share the same symptom complex and signs as cerebral infarcts except that early decrease in level of consciousness, nausea and vomiting, headache, and accelerated hypertension are more common with hemorrhages.

Subarachnoid hemorrhages classically present as a bursting very severe headache ("the worst headache of my life"), and are often accompanied by stiff neck, decreased consciousness, nausea and vomiting. Focal neurological signs are often absent; if present, they usually signify associated bleeding into the parenchyma.

Signs and symptoms characteristic of the various arterial territories

- Middle cerebral – contralateral loss of strength and sensation in the face, arm, and to a lesser extent leg. Aphasia if dominant hemisphere, neglect if non-dominant.
- Anterior cerebral – contralateral loss of strength and sensation in the leg and to a lesser extent arm.
- Posterior cerebral – contralateral visual field deficit. Possibly confusion and aphasia if dominant hemisphere.
- Penetrating (lacunar syndrome) – contralateral weakness or sensory loss (usually not both) in face, arm, and leg. No aphasia, neglect, or visual loss. Possibly ataxia, dysarthria.
- Vertebral (or posterior inferior cerebellar) – truncal ataxia, dysarthria, dysphagia, ipsilateral sensory loss on the face, and contralateral sensory loss below the neck.
- Basilar – various combinations of limb ataxia, dysarthria, dysphagia, facial and limb weakness and sensory loss (may be bilateral), pupillary asymmetry, disconjugate gaze, visual field loss, decreased responsiveness.

DIAGNOSIS

There is currently no 100% sensitive and specific test for cerebral infarction in the emergency department, so that the diagnosis is usually made on the basis of a characteristic history, exam, presence of comorbidities, and the absence of seizures or other stroke mimics. CT scanning is usually negative in the first three hours, or shows only subtle signs that have low inter-observer reliability. If available, MR imaging, or detection of an occluded artery by transcranial Doppler or arteriography (by CT, MRI or intra-arterial catheterization), can be confirmatory. Parenchymal or subarachnoid hemorrhage, on the other hand, can be reliably detected by emergent CT scanning.

STROKE MIMICS

All of the following may present similarly to a stroke. In all cases, the distinction can be made by an emergent MRI scan, which will show abnormal diffusion-weighted signal in most stroke cases, but not in mimics.

- Seizures. If a seizure has a focal onset in the brain, the patient may be left with weakness, numbness, speech, or vision problems for a period of time (usually less than 24 hours) after the seizure. Unlike the typical cerebral infarct, focal deficits after a seizure are often accompanied by lethargy and have a resolving course, but if the patient has had a seizure accompanying a stroke it is impossible to know for sure how much of the deficit the patient displays is due to each. This is why patients with seizures at onset are usually excluded from clinical trials of new stroke therapies.

- Migraine. Patients may have unilateral weakness or numbness, visual changes, or speech disturbances associated with a migraine headache ("complicated" or "complex" migraine). Also, patients with complicated migraine are at higher risk for stroke. In trying to make the distinction between complicated migraine and stroke, it is important to remember that because of the high prevalence of both migraine and stroke in the general population, it is dangerous to attribute the patient's deficit to migraine just because the patient has a migraine history. The best rule of thumb is not to make the diagnosis of complicated migraine or migrainous stroke unless the patient has a history of previous complicated migraine events similar to the deficit displayed in the emergency department.

- Syncope. This is usually due to hypotension or a cardiac arrhythmia. Stroke rarely presents with syncope alone. Patients with vertebrobasilar insufficiency may have syncope, but there are usually other brainstem or cerebellar findings if syncope is part of the stroke presentation.
- Hypoglycemia. Patients with low blood sugar may have symptoms that exactly mimic a stroke. The important thing is to check the blood sugar and, if low, correct it. If the symptoms do not resolve with correction of the hypoglycemia, the symptoms are probably from a stroke.
- Metabolic encephalopathy. Patients may have confusion, slurred speech, or rarely aphasia with this condition. They usually do not have other prominent focal findings.
- Drug overdose. Similar to metabolic encephalopathy.
- Central nervous system tumor. The location of the tumor would determine the type of signs and symptoms seen. A tumor, unlike a stroke, usually does not present with sudden focal findings, unless accompanied by a seizure (see above).
- Herpes simplex encephalitis (HSE). This infection tends predominantly to affect the temporal lobes, so patients may have signs of aphasia, hemiparesis or visual-field cuts. Onset can be rapid and in its early stages may mimic a stroke, but fever,

CSF pleocytosis, seizures and decreased level of consciousness are more prominent with HSE.

- Subdural hematoma. Depending on the location, this may cause contralateral weakness or numbness that may mimic a stroke. A CT scan can make this diagnosis, but the subdural, if small, may be subtle.
- Peripheral compression neuropathy. This may cause weakness or numbness in a particular peripheral nerve distribution and is usually not sudden in onset.
- Bell's palsy (peripheral seventh nerve palsy). The important point here is that the forehead and eye closure are weak on the same side. One can have a stroke involving the pons and produce a peripheral seventh nerve palsy, but usually there are other signs and symptoms such as weakness, a gaze palsy, or ipsilateral sixth nerve palsy.
- Benign paroxysmal positional vertigo (BPPV). This may cause vertigo, nausea, vomiting, and a sense of imbalance, usually with turning of the head in one direction. This characteristic syndrome is due to labyrinthine dysfunction and not stroke. However, as with syncope, the presence of any brainstem or cerebellar signs should alert one to the possibility of a stroke.
- Conversion disorder. Patients may develop neurological signs or symptoms of weakness, numbness, or trouble talking that are manifestations of stress or a psychiatric illness. Always assume that your patient has a true neurologic illness first.

■ What type of stroke?

As discussed previously, there are two main types of stroke: ischemic and hemorrhagic. The majority of this book describes the approach to either type of stroke, but there are specific chapters on ischemic stroke, TIA, ICH, and SAH:

- Ischemic stroke (Chapter 3).
- Transient ischemic attack (Chapter 7).
- Intracerebral hemorrhage (Chapter 8).
- Subarachnoid hemorrhage (Chapter 9).

2

What to do first

The following initial measures apply to all stroke patients. They are necessary to stabilize and assess the patient, and prepare for definitive therapy. All current and, probably, future stroke therapies for both ischemic and hemorrhagic stroke are best implemented as fast as possible, so these things need to be done quickly. This is the general order to do things, but in reality, in order to speed the process, these measures are usually dealt with simultaneously. They are best addressed in the ED, where urgent care pathways for stroke should be established and part of the routine (see Chapter 10).

■ Airway – breathing – circulation (ABCs)

- O_2 via nasal cannula (routine oxygen delivery in ischemia might improve outcome).*
- Intubation may be necessary if the patient shows arterial oxygen desaturation or cannot "protect" their airway from aspirating secretions. However, intubation means that the ability to monitor the neurological exam is lost. The best approach in such patients is to prepare to intubate immediately, but before doing so, take a moment to be sure the patient does not spontaneously improve or stabilize with

good nursing care (suctioning, head position, etc.). Also, if needed, use sedating or paralyzing drugs with a short half-life, to allow for serial neurological exams.

- Consider putting the head of the bed flat. This can significantly help cerebral perfusion. The head of the bed may need to be elevated if airway protection and continued nausea and vomiting are concerns for those with obtundation, nausea, severe dysphagia, or aspiration risk.
- Consider normal saline bolus 250–500 cc if blood pressure is low.
- If the blood pressure is high, antihypertensive treatment is discussed in subsequent chapters (Chapters 3, 4, 5, and 8).

■ What was the time of onset?

- Determining the exact time of onset is critical for establishing eligibility for acute therapies, especially TPA (Chapter 4). It is very important to be a detective. You will usually be told a time by the paramedics or ED triage nurse, but be sure to recheck the information you receive from them. If possible, try to speak personally with first-hand witnesses, nursing home staff, etc. Often paramedic information is based on an inexact estimate given to the paramedic when they arrive on scene, and then gets handed down as fact. You can often help establish the time of onset by finding out the time that the emergency call arrived at the dispatch center, and work backwards with the person who called. Other useful questions are to remind bystanders of their daily routine, TV shows, etc. that might help them accurately establish the time they found the patient or called the emergency services.
- In most cases, the onset is not observed – the patient is found with the deficit. In that case, or in patients who awaken

with symptoms, the onset time is the time the patient was last seen normal. However, if the patient awoke with symptoms, be sure to ask if the patient was up in the middle of the night for any reason (often to go to the bathroom) – as sometimes this puts the patient in the time window for treatment.

■ How bad are the symptoms now?

- Examine the patient and do the NIH stroke scale (NIHSS) (Appendix 14).
- The initial stroke severity is the most important predictor of outcome.

■ Do a non-contrast head CT

- This will immediately rule out hemorrhage (Chapters 8, 9) as blood is bright on a CT. The initial head CT should not show obvious acute ischemic changes in patients with ischemic infarcts who are eligible for acute interventions (Chapters 3–7), as acute ischemic changes become increasingly apparent between 3 and 24 hours.
- The result will determine the first major branching point in therapeutic decision-making, to be covered in the subsequent chapters.
- Obtaining the CT is often the major impediment in preparing for thrombolytic therapy, so efforts should be made to shorten "door to CT" time, which should be below 30 minutes. For instance, we allow the triage nurse to order the CT scan if a stroke is suspected, and stroke patients will get preference over any other patient for CT access. Another problem is prompt reading of CT scans, especially in small hospitals in

rural communities. Make sure to notify the reading radiologist that this patient is a possible TPA candidate.
- In some select centers, emergent MRI can be done very quickly and substitute for CT, but this is the exception. In general, MRI is deferred until after the first decision is made whether to treat with TPA.

■ If the CT shows no blood, try to get the artery open

- TPA is the only FDA-approved treatment for ischemic stroke, and you should immediately begin to determine if the patient is eligible for this therapy, and prepare for its administration. The TPA protocol is detailed in Chapter 4.

■ Recommended diagnostic evaluation

- The American Stroke Association guidelines list the following diagnostic studies for immediate use in a patient with suspected acute ischemic stroke.[1,2] These should be ordered in the ED, but you should not delay TPA treatment waiting for results once the patient meets established criteria (Chapter 4).

All patients
- brain CT (brain MRI could be considered at qualified centers)
- electrocardiogram
- blood glucose
- serum electrolytes
- renal function tests

- complete blood count, including platelet count
- prothrombin time/international normalized ratio
- activated partial thromboplastin time

Selected patients
- hepatic function tests
- toxicology screen
- blood alcohol determination
- pregnancy test
- oxygen saturation or arterial blood gas tests (if hypoxia is suspected)
- chest radiography (if lung disease or aortic dissection are suspected)
- lumbar puncture (if subarachnoid hemorrhage is suspected and CT is negative for blood)
- electroencephalogram (if seizures are suspected)

3

Ischemic stroke

This chapter discusses the four main components of acute ischemic stroke care. The sections on prevention of complications and recovery and rehabilitation are applicable to both ischemic and hemorrhagic stroke patients.

■ Definition

An ischemic stroke is death of brain tissue due to interruption of blood flow to a region of the brain, caused by occlusion of a cerebral or cervical artery or, less likely, a cerebral vein.

■ Etiology

The etiology of the ischemic stroke is important to help determine the best treatment to prevent another stroke. However, regardless of etiology, initial therapy is for the most part the same, and so initially, the most important thing is to implement the acute measures described in this chapter.

■ Diagnosis

The first important task is to differentiate between ischemic and hemorrhagic stroke, which can be done with a head CT. Detailed brain and vascular imaging are critically important but should not delay assessment for TPA candidacy. There are things that can mimic stroke (see Chapter 1).

A focused history should quickly exclude stroke mimics. Unless the presentation is atypical or a stroke mimic is suggested, one should assume it is a stroke and proceed with the determination of whether or not the patient is a candidate for acute therapy. A detailed diagnostic evaluation should be deferred.

■ The four components of ischemic stroke care

There are four components to caring for people with acute ischemic stroke. At every point, you should be thinking about the four issues:

(1) Acute therapy and optimization of neurological status.
(2) Etiological work-up for secondary prevention.
(3) Prevention of neurological deterioration or medical complications.
(4) Recovery and rehabilitation.

This chapter discusses the four components in brief, and then there are longer discussions on the following topics:

• TPA therapy (Chapter 4).
• Neurological deterioration (Chapter 5).
• Stroke prevention (Chapter 6).
• Rehabilitation (Chapter 11).

See also the sample admission orders in Appendix 3.

■ Acute therapy and optimization of neurological status

The main goal of therapy is to get the artery open and re-establish blood flow. You should always ask yourself if you

are doing everything possible to optimize blood flow to regions of cerebral ischemia.

INTRAVENOUS RECOMBINANT TISSUE PLASMINOGEN ACTIVATOR (TPA)

In this book, we will refer to recombinant tissue plasminogen activator as TPA, because that is what it is usually called in the busy emergency department. However, the reader should be aware that this drug is also referred to as rt-PA, t-PA, tPA, alteplase (generic name) or Activase (trade name).

- Intravenous TPA is the only FDA-approved treatment for ischemic stroke in the USA. It is approved under safety monitoring in the European Union. Intra-arterial (IA) thrombolysis is a rescue therapy that is being used in several centers under various research protocols. A variety of neuroprotective agents (hypothermia, other drugs) are presently under investigation to try to decrease infarct size, but none is FDA-approved at this time.
- The current guideline is that TPA should be given if the patient meets criteria for treatment.[2] Details of the protocol can be found in Chapter 4.

CONCURRENT DIAGNOSTIC TESTING

Determination of stroke etiology is usually deferred until after starting TPA therapy. However, while considering or instituting TPA, concomitant information about vascular and tissue status may be helpful. For instance, detection of large-artery occlusion or stenosis is particularly helpful in planning acute recanalization strategies and risk stratification for recurrent stroke or neurological deterioration.

The following diagnostic tests may be helpful in determining the stroke mechanism, however, the need to do acute studies depends on a balance of availability of therapy, time requirement, clinical suspicion, and cost.

- Head CT should already have been done, as it is one of the vital first steps in the management of the stroke patient and helps to exclude hemorrhage (see Chapter 2).
- Transcranial Doppler ultrasound (TCD) can be performed to detect occlusion, recanalization, and reocclusion of the large intracranial arteries in real time and can be brought to the patient's bedside in the emergency department.
- CT angiography (CTA) can quickly provide a snapshot of the entire cerebral arterial anatomy, and can diagnose intracranial and extracranial stenoses, aneurysms, or dissections. It is important to know the patient's creatinine prior to the administration of IV contrast and exclude a contrast allergy.
- MR angiography (MRA) of the neck and circle of Willis provides the same information as CTA without risk of contrast. However, patients must be cooperative to hold still for several minutes, and those with a pacemaker and some with aneurysm clips or stents may not be eligible for MRI scanning.
- MR imaging (MRI) of the brain can provide substantial information on stroke localization, age, bleeding, and tissue status (see Appendix 5). However, the same caveats apply as with MRA.

MAINTENANCE OF CEREBRAL PERFUSION

To maximize brain perfusion through stenoses and collateral vessels, we maintain euvolemia, support blood pressure, and put the head of the bed flat.

Do not treat hypertension acutely* unless:

(1) the patient was treated with TPA*

    or

(2) the patient has acute hypertensive end organ damage (congestive heart failure, myocardial infarction, hypertensive encephalopathy, dissecting aortic aneurysm, etc.)*

    or

(3) systolic or diastolic pressures are above 220 or 120 mm Hg respectively*

If you are going to treat hypertension, consider using a short-acting agent that will wear off quickly or be turned off in case BP drops too much, such as:

- labetalol (Trandate, Normodyne) 10–20 mg IV*
- nicardipine (Cardene) 5 mg/hr IV infusion as initial dose; titrate to desired effect by increasing 2.5 mg/hr every 5 minutes to maximum of 15 mg/hr*

Goal: Blood pressure reduction by 10–15%.

See Table 3.1 for current guidelines on the treatment of hypertension in acute ischemic stroke. In the absence of controlled prospective data, there is some consensus but still significant uncertainty about what levels of blood pressure to treat, how fast to lower the pressure, and what drugs to use. In acute ischemic stroke, we follow the guidelines in Table 3.1; we use nicardipine most commonly in the ED and during the first 24 hours to titrate blood pressure smoothly to desired levels.

Other options for maintenance of cerebral perfusion

- Normal saline for IV fluids – to maintain euvolemia and because it is isotonic and will not cause fluid shifts:
  - consider normal saline 500 cc bolus over 20–30 minutes.
- Consider hetastarch (Hespan, Hextend) for volume expansion:
  - hetastarch 500 cc over 1 hour;

Table 3.1. Approach to elevated blood pressure in acute ischemic stroke.

Blood Pressure Level (mm Hg)	Treatment
A. Not eligible for thrombolytic therapy	
Systolic < 220 OR Diastolic < 120	Observe unless other end-organ involvement, e.g., aortic dissection, acute myocardial infarction, pulmonary edema, hypertensive encephalopathy
	Treat other symptoms of stroke such as headache, pain, agitation, nausea, and vomiting
	Treat other acute complication of stroke, including hypoxia, increased intracranial pressure, seizures, or hypoglycemia
Systolic > 220 OR Diastolic < 121–140	Labetalol 10–20 mg IV over 1–2 min May repeat or double every 10 min (maximum dose 300 mg) or Nicardipine 5 mg/hr IV infusion as initial dose; titrate to desired effect by increasing 2.5 mg/hr every 5 min to maximum of 15 mg/hr Aim for a 10% to 15% reduction of blood pressure
Diastolic > 140	Nitroprusside 0.5 µg/kg/min IV infusion as initial dose with continuous blood pressure monitoring Aim for a 10% to 15% reduction of blood pressure
B. Eligible for thrombolytic therapy	
Pretreatment	
Systolic > 185 OR Diastolic > 110	Labetalol 10–20 mg IV over 1–2 min May repeat × 1 OR Nitropaste 1–2 inches If blood pressure is not reduced and maintained at desired levels (systolic ≤ 185 and diastolic ≤ 110), do not administer TPA

Table 3.1. (*cont.*)

Blood Pressure Level (mm Hg)	Treatment
During and after treatment	
1. Monitor BP	Check BP every 15 min for 2 hours, then every 30 min for 6 hours, and then every hour for 16 hours
2. Diastolic > 140	Sodium nitroprusside 0.5 μg/kg/min IV infusion as initial dose and titrate to desired blood pressure
3. Systolic > 230 OR Diastolic 121–140	Labetalol 10 mg IV over 1–2 min
	May repeat or double labetalol every 10 min to a maximum dose of 300 mg or give the initial labetalol bolus and then start a labetalol drip at 2 to 8 mg/min
	or
	Nicardipine 5 mg/hr IV infusion as initial dose; Titrate to desired effect by increasing 2.5 mg/hr every 5 min to maximum of 15 mg/hr. If BP is not controlled by labetalol, consider sodium nitroprusside
4. Systolic 180–230 OR Diastolic 105–120	Labetalol 10 mg IV over 1–2 min
	May repeat or double labetalol every 10 to 20 min to a maximum dose of 300 mg or give the initial labetalol bolus and then start a labetalol drip at 2 to 8 mg/min

Source: H. P. Adams Jr., R. J. Adams, T. Brott, *et al.*, Guidelines for the early management of patients with ischemic stroke: a scientific statement from the Stroke Council of the American Stroke Association. *Stroke* 2003; **34**: 1056–83.[1] Reproduced with permission from Lippincott Williams & Wilkins.

- then consider hetastarch 250 cc IV every 8 hours. Monitor jugular venous pressure and input/output. Watch for fluid overload.
- Consider phenylephrine (Neo-Synephrine) drip, or other pressors, in ICU for induced hypertension.

ANTIPLATELET AND ANTICOAGULANT THERAPY AS AN ACUTE TREATMENT FOR ISCHEMIC STROKE

Both antiplatelet and anticoagulant therapy are often considered in the acute therapy of ischemic stroke, and one or both may be appropriate, but randomized trials have shown that anticoagulants should not be routinely employed acutely. Trials have shown that antiplatelets have only a modest benefit, and no studies have yet shown the benefit of urgent antiplatelet treatment.

Acute antiplatelet therapy

Aspirin for acute stroke has been shown to be effective, though only marginally, when studied in thousands of patients.[3,4*]

Antiplatelet treatment beyond aspirin is driven by evidence from acute cardiovascular trials until there are more stroke data available, remembering of course the greater propensity of the brain to develop hemorrhagic complications.

We give aspirin 81–325 mg to most patients. In patients who have had strokes or TIAs while already on antiplatelet therapy, who have a fluctuating neurological course, or who have a heavy burden of atherosclerotic risk factors or atherosclerotic lesions, we will often orally load the patient in the emergency department with clopidogrel (Plavix) 375 mg, and then aspirin 81 mg and clopidogrel 75 mg once daily for the first few days. The idea of an oral load stems from studies in patients undergoing coronary procedures who have less peri-procedural ischemic complications if they receive a load pre-procedure. We then switch to aspirin/dipyridamole combination (Aggrenox, Asasantin)* or aspirin alone* or clopidogrel alone* if the patient is going home on antiplatelets.

Acute anticoagulant therapy

Anticoagulation for acute ischemic stroke has never been shown to be effective.[3*] Even among those with atrial fibrillation, the stroke recurrence rate is only ~5–8% in the first 14 days, which is not reduced by early acute anticoagulation.[5,6*] Anticoagulation is mostly used for long-term secondary prevention in patients with atrial fibrillation and cardioembolic stroke at this point.

   Without convincing supporting data, some clinicians advocate acute anticoagulation with heparin in certain cases. These include patients with a cardioembolic condition at high risk for recurrence (thrombus on valves, or mural thrombus), documented large-artery (ICA, MCA, or basilar artery) occlusive clot at risk for distal embolism, arterial dissection, or venous thrombosis. Such patients may be started on heparin acutely and transitioned to warfarin (Coumadin). If ordering heparin, use weight-adjusted algorithm with **no** bolus*. Enoxaparin (Lovenox) at 1 mg/kg subcutaneously every 12 hours may be used in place of heparin.

   How long should you wait before starting anticoagulation? There are no clear data on this topic. There is concern that the risk of hemorrhagic conversion is increased with anticoagulation, particularly in patients with large strokes. Hemorrhagic transformation is frequent in the evolution of large infarcts, especially those that have been reperfused either by spontaneous recanalization or with thrombolytics. One should be particularly careful about early anticoagulation in these patients. One generally waits 2–14 days before starting anticoagulation, the specific duration depending on the urgency of the indication versus the risks. You must carefully weigh the risks and benefits on a case by case basis, and **never start anticoagulants without obtaining brain imaging first**, to exclude ongoing hemorrhagic evolution or brain swelling.

HYPERGLYCEMIA

Hyperglycemia is known to worsen stroke outcome. The mechanism by which and level at which hyperglycemia worsens stroke is not known. However, there are data that show even modest hyperglycemia (glucose > 150 mg/dl) enlarges eventual stroke size and increases the risk of brain hemorrhage. Therefore, **treat glucose aggressively**.

See Appendix 8 for insulin algorithm.

HYPERTHERMIA

Hyperthermia has been correlated with poor outcome. Experimentally, increasing the body temperature of animals increases metabolic demand and infarct size. Therefore, treat hyperthermia aggressively with acetaminophen (Tylenol) and cooling blankets if necessary.*

■ Etiological work-up for secondary prevention

See also Chapter 6, which covers in more detail the evaluation of stroke patients and how to choose secondary prevention strategies in relation to the results of the diagnostic considerations.

With brain imaging and vascular evaluation we try to find a **specific etiology** such as cardioembolic source, arterial stenosis, etc. (Fig. 3.1). At the same time, we look for reversible **risk factors** for recurrent stroke such as hypertension, diabetes, hypercholesterolemia, and smoking/substance abuse that will need to be addressed.

There are several different ways to classify strokes (based on severity, location, size, etc.), but for planning a secondary stroke prevention strategy we find the following TOAST classification[8] most useful, since it is based on stroke mechanism.

- Large-artery atherosclerosis: intracranial, extracranial (carotid, aortic arch).
- Cardioembolic: atrial fibrillation, segmental wall akinesis, paradoxical embolus, etc.
- Small vessel: lacunar infarction.
- Other: unusual causes (dissection, venous thrombosis, drugs, etc.).
- Unknown: cryptogenic.

SCREENING FOR ARTERIAL STENOSIS/OBSTRUCTION

MR angiography (**MRA**) shows arterial stenosis intracranially and extracranially, and excludes large aneurysms and vascular malformations. It is a good screening tool. Recent data indicate that **contrast-enhanced MRA** might be the most reliable of non-invasive tests.[9] In our hands, **carotid ultrasound** is better at estimating the degree of internal carotid artery (ICA) stenosis at the bifurcation. **TCD** complements other vascular imaging and can also be used to follow changes over time.

You will often focus on the origins of the internal carotid arteries, but do not forget the vertebral artery origins and

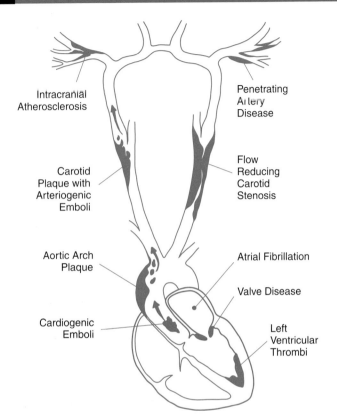

Figure 3.1. Mechanisms of stroke.
Source: G. W. Albers, P. Amarenco, J. D. Easton, R. L. Sacco, & P. Teal,
Antithrombotic and thrombolytic therapy for ischemic stroke: the Seventh
ACCP Conference on Antithrombotic and Thrombolytic Therapy. *Chest* 2004;
126 (3 suppl.): 483S–512S.[7] Reproduced with permission.

intracranial arteries that often harbor atherosclerotic narrowing which may be the etiology of the stroke.

Digital subtraction angiography (**DSA**) is considered the gold standard for visualizing the arteries, but is not without risk.

CT angiography can give you sufficient detail and can be done quickly from the ED. DSA often takes much longer to obtain due to the need to organize the angiography team. For determining degree of arterial stenoses, seeing arterial dissection, or other vascular abnormalities, however, DSA is still considered the gold standard.

CARDIAC EVALUATION

An **electrocardiogram** (**EKG**) should be done to exclude atrial fibrillation and to rule out silent myocardial infarction or ischemia, which may occur as a consequence of the stroke. If atrial fibrillation or other important arrhythmia is suspected, cardiac telemetry or Holter monitor is needed.

An **echocardiogram** is helpful in looking for a cardioembolic source and right-to-left shunts. A **transthoracic echocardiogram** (**TTE**) can show wall motion abnormalities (anterior wall akinesis carries high embolic risk), low left ventricular ejection fraction (<20–30% generally agreed upon as a cutoff), valvular abnormalities, and a patent foramen ovale (PFO).

Transesophageal echocardiogram (**TEE**) can show the atria better. Left atrial appendage clot, size of PFO, PFO associated with atrial septal aneurysm, aortic arch atheroma, and spontaneous echo contrast are some of the findings associated with increased risk for ischemic stroke. Long-term anticoagulation with warfarin is considered to be the best prevention strategy for cardioembolic sources, but for many of the etiologies, it is still controversial whether warfarin is better than antiplatelets.

TCD with bubble contrast is as sensitive as TEE for detection of right-to-left shunt.

RECURRENT STROKE RISK FACTOR SCREENING

- Monitor blood pressure.*
- Obtain fasting lipid panel.*
- Screen for diabetes.
- Screen for hyperhomocysteinemia (though a risk factor, whether or not screening and therapy are beneficial is controversial).
- Smoking cessation counseling, if applicable.*

■ Prevention of neurological deterioration or medical complications

Neurological deterioration and medical complications will be covered in more detail in Chapter 5 and Appendix 9.

THE FOLLOWING MEASURES SHOULD BE INSTITUTED IN ALL STROKE PATIENTS

- Deep venous thrombosis (DVT) prophylaxis (pharmacologic, devices, patient mobilization).
- Aspiration precautions (swallowing assessment and nursing supervision before allowing the patient to eat).
- Gastrointestinal ulcer prophylaxis.
- Take out indwelling urinary (Foley) catheter as soon as possible.
- Monitor platelet counts if on heparin to watch for heparin-induced thrombocytopenia (HIT).

THE FOLLOWING ISSUES MUST BE ADDRESSED DAILY

- Is the patient neurologically stable or improving?
  - Avoid dehydration of dysphagic patients with limited oral intake.
  - Avoid diuretics in patients receiving IV fluids.
- Is the patient medically stable (e.g., congestive heart failure, infection)?
- Is the blood pressure coming down slowly?
- Is the patient eating safely?
- Is the patient comfortable and sleeping well?
  - Ask yourself why the patient *still* gets blood drawn every morning for blood count, chemistry, calcium . . .
- What is the mechanism of the stroke?
  - Is the work-up appropriate and complete?
- What are we doing to prevent another stroke?
- Ask yourself why the patient is *not* on antiplatelets, statins, ACE inhibitors – because most patients on the stroke service should be (except people with ICH or on anticoagulation).
- What are we doing to promote recovery?
- What are we doing to prevent complications from the stroke?
  - Don't forget DVT prophylaxis.
  - Ask yourself why the patient still has a Foley catheter and IV fluids if the patient is being discharged soon.
- What is the disposition?
- Think about disposition early:
  - Consult physical therapy, occupational therapy and rehabilitation.
  - Contact primary care provider for follow-up.
  - Arrange home health care if indicated.

DRUG THERAPY IN THE FIRST 72 HOURS

(those most commonly started in our stroke unit)

Antiplatelets
- Aspirin 81–325 mg once daily*, or
- Clopidogrel (Plavix) 75 mg PO once daily*, or
- Aspirin 25 mg/dipyridamole 200 mg extended release (Aggrenox/Asasantin) twice daily.*

DVT prophylaxis
- Heparin 5000 units SC every 12 hours*, or
- Enoxaparin (Lovenox, Clexane) 40 mg SC once daily, or
- Dalteparin (Fragmin) 5000 units SC once daily;
- Sequential compression devices (non-drug);
- Compression (TED) stockings.

Anticoagulants for cardioembolic stroke
- Weight-adjusted heparin (see Appendix 7).
- Warfarin (Coumadin) (start with 5–10 mg day).*

Insulin if needed (see Appendix 8)*

Temperature control with acetaminophen if needed*

HMG CoA reductase inhibitors with goal of LDL < 100*

Oral antihypertensive agents*
- ACE inhibitors:
  - Lisinopril (Prinivil, Zestril) 10–40 mg daily.
  - Perindopril (Aceon, Coversyl) 4 mg PO once daily.
  - Ramipril (Altace) starting at 2.5–5 mg daily; target 10 mg PO once daily.

- Angiotensin receptor blockers (ARBs):
  - Losartan (Cozaar) 25–100 mg daily.
- Diuretics:
  - Hydrochlorothiazide (HCTZ), chlorthalidone (Hygroton) 25 mg daily.
- Beta-blockers:
  - Metoprolol (Lopressor, Toprol) 25–450 mg daily.
- Calcium channel blockers:
  - Amlodipine (Norvasc) 5–10 mg daily.

■ Stroke recovery and rehabilitation

See also Chapter 10 (Organization of stroke care) and Chapter 11 (Rehabilitation).

Physical therapy (PT), occupational therapy (OT), and speech pathology should get involved *early*!*

Patients who are eating (after swallowing assessment by speech pathology) are happy patients, and this also makes family members happy. The sooner you get the patient and family involved in the process of recovery and rehabilitation the earlier you will be able to begin working on placement at the appropriate location (home, rehabilitation, skilled nursing facility (SNF), nursing home, or long-term acute care facility [LTAC]). The **rehabilitation team** is the key to determining disposition.

The only times when PT/OT would not be involved early is when the patient is obtunded or needs to lie flat in bed in an attempt to maximize cerebral perfusion. It is very important to get the patient mobilized with an out-of-bed (OOB) order (e.g., out of bed with meals, with PT, etc.). Mobilization also prevents complications.

■ Ischemic stroke outcome

Outcome after stroke depends on stroke severity, size, mechanism, age, premorbid functional status, whether and when the patient received TPA, and whether the patient is cared for in a stroke unit.

MORTALITY

Overall (data from Rochester Epidemiology Project and NOMASS):[10,11]

- ~30% mortality in the first year.
- 40–50% in 5 years.

From Medicare database (age $\geq$ 65 years):[12]

- After surviving an **ischemic stroke** hospitalization, **26.4% mortality** in 1 year, 60% mortality after 5 years.
- After surviving a **TIA** hospitalization, **15% mortality** in 1 year, 50% mortality in 5 years.

DISABILITY

More importantly than mortality, patients and families usually are anxious to know their likely functional outcome. This is very difficult to predict in the first few days in an individual patient. It is best to offer a range from "worst case" to "best case" scenarios.

Table 3.2 shows outcome data based on ischemic stroke subtype as determined by the extent of arterial occlusion, i.e., total, partial, or lacunar.

Table 3.2. Ischemic stroke outcomes from a population-based study in Australia.

	Dead	Disabled	Non-disabled	Alive, not assessed
Total anterior circulation infarction (TACI)				
3 months	56%	29%	0%	15%
1 year	62%	24%	3%	12%
Partial anterior circulation infarction (PACI)				
3 months	13%	36%	24%	28%
1 year	25%	29%	24%	22%
Posterior circulation infarction (POCI)				
3 months	16%	20%	27%	38%
1 year	24%	22%	22%	31%
Lacunar infarction (LACI)				
3 months	8%	24%	31%	37%
1 year	8%	24%	31%	37%
Total				
3 months	20%	29%	22%	30%
1 year	31%	23%	23%	23%

Source: H. M. Dewey, J. Sturm, G. A. Donnan, R. A. Macdonell, J. J. McNeil, & A. G. Thrift, Incidence and outcome of subtypes of ischaemic stroke: initial results from the North East Melbourne stroke incidence study (NEMESIS). *Cerebrovasc. Dis.* 2003; **15**: 133–9.[13] Reproduced with permission from S. Karger AG, Basel.

AT PATIENT DISCHARGE

Be sure you have determined or done the following:
- What is the stroke location and mechanism?
- What strategies are we using to prevent another stroke?

- Is the patient on any antihypertensives, in particular ACE inhibitor?
- Is the patient on antiplatelets (e.g., aspirin, aspirin/ dipyridamole, or clopidogrel)?
- Is the patient's LDL < 100 mg/dl and is he or she on a statin?
- Get rid of unnecessary drugs.
- Is the follow-up plan established? If the patient is discharged on warfarin, who will be following the INR? This is critically important to communicate to the primary care providers as they are the ones who will be managing the risk factors of anticoagulation on a long-term basis.
- It is important to convey the mechanism of stroke and treatment recommendations to the primary care provider who will assume the primary responsibility for management of the patient on discharge.
- Dictate a discharge summary that includes the above thought processes (see Appendix 4 for sample).

■ General timeline

The following is a general timeline for the care of stroke patients. It is affected by the severity of the stroke, extent of diagnostic work-up necessary to determine etiology, ability to swallow, and amount of early recovery. The goal is to get patients discharged from acute hospitalization as quickly and as safely as possible.

- Stroke unit for 1–3 days.
- Then to the general ward to finish work-up and disposition determination.
- Discharge by day 2–5.

4

TPA protocol

Intravenous TPA is the only FDA-approved therapy for acute ischemic stroke, based on the pivotal NINDS TPA Stroke Study.[14*] The drug is now approved in North America, Europe, and Japan for treating acute ischemic stroke. In the USA, IV TPA has been utilized for over a decade, and numerous meta-analyses and post-marketing studies confirm that, if guidelines [1,2] are adhered to, there are substantial benefits and the risks are minimized. On the other hand, if these are violated, then the risks begin to outweigh the benefits.

Having given this cautionary statement, there is some variability in how strictly the published exclusion criteria are applied in practice at our own center. For the most part, the following indications and contraindications follow published guidelines.[1,2] We have indicated beneath each guideline where we might allow some flexibility in interpreting these criteria.

■ TPA indications

- Age 18 or older – There are no data to guide treatment in children. However, there are case reports of older children being treated with TPA using adult criteria.
- Clinical diagnosis of ischemic stroke causing a measurable neurological deficit – Stroke must be of more than minimal

severity (in almost all cases, NIH stroke scale score ≥ 3). We use the criterion, "Would it be disabling if the deficit were to persist?"

- Onset of stroke symptoms well established to be less than 180 minutes (3 hours) before treatment would begin – We have addressed the importance of establishing the time of onset in Chapter 2.

■ Strong contraindications

- Symptoms minor or rapidly improving – This is one of the most difficult decisions in treating patients with TPA. Guidelines state not to treat a patient who is rapidly improving. However, we have found that many such patients recover substantially but are still left with a disabling deficit. Even patients with very mild strokes benefit from TPA treatment, and intracranial bleeding complications in such patients are very rare. Therefore, instead of automatically excluding all patients who are improving or have minor deficits, we would still treat the minor or improving patient whose deficit, at the time you are ready to treat, would be disabling if it persisted.
- Known history of intracranial hemorrhage.
- Symptoms suggestive of subarachnoid hemorrhage.
- Any evidence of bleeding on the pretreatment head CT – It is uncertain whether patients with "microbleeds" that are seen on gradient echo MRI (and not CT) can be safely treated. Most recent data suggest that they do not pose an increased risk of bleeding after TPA, but the data are still inconclusive. However, if there is **any** bleeding seen on the CT, the patient should not be treated.
- Intracranial neoplasm, untreated arteriovenous malformation (AVM), or aneurysm that is at risk of bleeding – If the patient

has an aneurysm or AVM that has been surgically clipped or repaired more than 3 months ago, we would probably allow treatment, though we would probably do a CT angiogram first to confirm obliteration of the lesion. Many patients with benign brain tumors such as meningiomas also have been treated without complications. However, patients with more aggressive brain tumors should not be treated.

- Significant hypodensity or mass effect on pretreatment CT – Early ischemic changes on the CT are not a contraindication. However, clearly demarcated hypodensity suggesting that the stroke is more than 3 hours old would argue against treatment. Mass effect with compression of the ventricle or midline structures would suggest a non-stroke etiology.
- Previous stroke, intracranial surgery, or serious head trauma within the past 3 months.
- Major surgery within the last 14 days.
- Sustained systolic blood pressure greater than 185 mm Hg.
- Sustained diastolic blood pressure greater than 110 mm Hg.
- Aggressive treatment necessary to lower blood pressure to these levels – See comments on blood-pressure control, below.
- Gastrointestinal or urinary tract hemorrhage within the last 21 days – In some cases, we are not so rigid with regard to time intervals for GI and GU bleeding, allowing for clinical judgment based on the severity of the anticipated risk vs. the possible benefit. For instance, one might be willing to treat a patient with a very severe stroke who has had some recent GI bleeding, knowing that they might have this complication, but also knowing that without treatment the outcome is likely to be very poor. This risk would be less acceptable in a patient with a milder stroke. The main caveat is that if the patient is actively bleeding, as evidenced by a low hemoglobin/hematocrit,

they should not be treated. If you do treat a patient with risk of bleeding, then consultation with the appropriate surgical consultant who could help manage the hemorrhagic complication should be obtained at the time of treatment, in anticipation of, and not after, the complication occurs.

- Arterial puncture at a noncompressible site or lumbar puncture – Guidelines state that TPA should not be given within 7 days of such punctures, but clinical judgment is necessary. Usually, 24 hours should be a sufficient interval if there is no evidence of an especially traumatic puncture.
- Received heparin within 48 hours *and* has an elevated PTT.
- Platelet count less than 100,000.
- INR greater than 1.7 or known bleeding diathesis – We are a little more conservative than published guidelines about the INR level that would allow treatment with IV TPA. In the NINDS trial, the cutoff used was a prothrombin time (PT) of 15 seconds. There is debate as to what INR level correlates with this level of PT. However, we know that increased bleeding occurs when patients treated with warfarin reach an INR of 1.7 or higher. For this reason we tend to be a little more conservative and use an INR cutoff of 1.6. We send patients with INRs above this level to intra-arterial mechanical clot removal (see below).

■ Relative contraindications

- Seizure at the onset of stroke – Patients with seizures were excluded from the initial studies of TPA because they made it difficult to assess how much of the neurologic deficit was due to the seizure and how much due to the stroke. This is important when carrying out a clinical trial, but less important in clinical practice. If you are sure that a stroke has occurred that is causing a disabling deficit, even if the patient has had a seizure, we feel it is appropriate to treat that patient if they qualify by other criteria (particularly no evidence of head trauma with the seizure).

- Blood glucose less than 50 mg/dL or greater than 400 mg/dL – If the patient remains symptomatic after a high or low glucose is treated and normalized, they need not be excluded.
- Hemorrhagic eye disorder, and other conditions likely to cause disability if bleeding occurs – Recent ocular surgery such as for cataracts, and other minor surgery, are not necessarily contra-indications. Judgment is needed. Treatment of a patient with some ocular conditions, such as a recently detached retina, might pose too great a risk of visual loss, especially if the stroke is relatively mild. The best course is to try to reach the specialist consultant and ask for an opinion about bleeding risk.
- Myocardial infarction in the prior 6 weeks – Again, judgment should be utilized in interpreting this exclusion. Both the time interval from the MI and the severity of the MI should be taken into consideration. The main risk here is hemorrhagic pericarditis and pericardial tamponade. This would certainly be a risk with a recent transmural MI or open-heart surgery, but a smaller MI, even if recent, would not be considered a contraindication.
- Suspected septic embolism or known infective endocarditis.

Blood pressure control is very important to prevent complications

Before treatment, the goal is <185/<110 mm Hg. **Labetalol** (Trandate, Normodyne) 10–20 mg IV or a **nicardipine** (Cardene) drip (start at 5 mg/h and titrate up to a maximum of 15 mg/h) may be given to lower the blood pressure. If you are unable to keep the BP in the specified range with

labetalol < 40 mg or nicardipine < 15 mg/h, the risk of hemorrhage is too high and the patient should not receive TPA.

■ Procedure

FAST!

Remember: time is brain. Best results occur with treatment
started within 2 hours of symptom onset.

- Check to make sure laboratory tests have been sent imme-
  diately and EKG ordered (ordered, drawn, and sent within the
  first 5 minutes).
  - Glucose, hemoglobin/hematocrit, and platelets are the only
    blood tests you need before treatment in most patients.
  - Glucose can be by fingerstick.
  - Complete blood count (CBC).
  - Coagulation studies (PTT, INR) if patient is on anticoagu-
    lants or coagulopathy is suspected.
  - Some centers now have a fingerstick INR.
  - Urine pregnancy test if appropriate.
- Examine patient (done within the next 5 minutes).
  - Establish clear time of onset.
  - Obtain pertinent historical details (e.g., past medical
    history, medications).
  - NIH stroke scale (Appendix 14).
- Obtain non-contrast head CT (maximum ED arrival to CT
  time should be 30 minutes).
- Talk to patient and family to explain risks/benefits.
- Obtain the patient's weight (ask the patient or family
  member(s), or estimate).
  - If the patient weighs over 100 kg (220 lb) they will get the
    maximum dose and it is not important to figure out the
    exact weight.

- Think again: go over indications/contraindications and lab and imaging results.
- Check BP again.
- Pre-therapy: 2 peripheral IV lines.
  - Foley catheter (optional).

Door to needle time: goal is <40 minutes, maximum is 60 minutes.

■ Dose

- TPA 0.9 mg/kg up to a maximum of 90 mg total.
- **10%** given as IV **bolus** over 1 minute.
- remaining **90% infused** over 1 hour.

Note: Only TPA has been approved for the treatment of stroke. **Other drugs** that may be given to patients with MI may **not be used** for stroke. These include reteplase (Retavase), tenecteplase (TNKase, Metalyse), streptokinase (Streptase). Make sure to double-check the name of the drug because there are some hospitals that may not carry TPA. ED personnel may reach for one of the other thrombolytic drugs due to their comfort with them for use in acute myocardial infarction. Also, the dosing for stroke and acute myocardial infarction are different.

■ Sample post-TPA orders

See Appendix 3.

TPA-RELATED INTRACRANIAL HEMORRHAGE: MANAGEMENT PROTOCOL

Stop TPA infusion if still running.

Goal: fibrinogen level > 100 mg/dL with cryoprecipitate.

- Type and cross.
- Check fibrinogen level immediately and every 6 hours.
- Give 10–20 units of cryoprecipitate before level returns (1 unit raises fibrinogen by 5–10 mg/dL; assume there is no fibrinogen and adjust dose when level is back).
- Repeat cryoprecipitate if needed.
- May use fresh frozen plasma (FFP) in case of no cryoprecipitate (1 unit of cryoprecipitate is made from 1 bag of FFP).
- May give platelet concentrate if low.
- Activated factor 7 is untested in this situation, and should not be used.
- Neurosurgery should be called; however, surgery cannot be done until coagulopathy is corrected and is usually not indicated.

OROPHARYNGEAL ANGIOEDEMA: MANAGEMENT PROTOCOL

- Repeatedly examine oropharynx, watching for edema (may be subtle swelling of lip or tongue just on one side).
- If angioedema is suspected, **immediately** call for personnel experienced in intubation and airway management. Do not wait until airway obstruction occurs.
- Choose from the following medication options:
  - Epinephrine 0.5 ml via nebulizer or 0.3 ml of 0.1% solution subcutaneously (may repeat 2 × as tolerated).
  - Diphenhydramine (Benadryl) 50 mg IV followed by 25 mg every 6 hours × 4 doses.
  - Methylprednisolone (Solumedrol) 100 mg IV; may follow with 20–80 mg IV daily for 3–5 days depending on degree and course of angioedema.
  - Famotidine 20 mg IV followed by 20 mg IV every 12 hours × 2 doses.

- If further increase in oropharyngeal angioedema is seen, or if there is airway compromise:
  - If tongue is edematous, but oral intubation is possible, perform urgent orotracheal intubation.
  - If tongue is too edematous for orotracheal intubation, perform fiberoptic nasotracheal intubation.
  - If there is severe stridor or impending airway obstruction, perform tracheostomy or cricothyrotomy and consider reversing TPA.
  - Always resolves spontaneously within 24 hours without sequelae.

■ Risks vs. benefits of TPA

WHAT ARE THE RISKS OF TPA THERAPY?

- Symptomatic intracranial hemorrhage rate 6.4% (i.e., 1 in 16; 95% CI 3.5–9.2%) vs. 0.6% in placebo.
- There have been cases of angioedema. In a retrospective series, it was reported to occur at a rate of 5.1% (95% CI 2.3–9.5%), but this is probably an overestimate (see above for treatment options). Occurs more frequently in patients taking angiotensin converting enzyme inhibitors.

WHAT ARE THE BENEFITS OF TPA THERAPY?

The percentage of patients with excellent outcome (Rankin 0–1) is increased by about 15% absolute, or 50% relative. The percentage with bad outcome (dead or Rankin 4–5) is reduced, even if you include the patients who bleed (Fig. 4.1).

Modified Rankin Scale

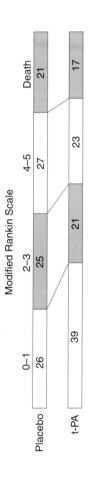

Percentage of Patients

Figure 4.1. Three-month outcome in NINDS TPA study by modified Rankin scale (see Appendix 14).

Source: The National Institute of Neurological Disorders and Stroke rt-PA Stroke Study Group, Tissue plasminogen activator for acute ischemic stroke. *N. Engl. J. Med.* 1995; **333**: 1581-7.[14] Reproduced with permission. Copyright © 1995 Massachusetts Medical Society.

- The odds ratio of good outcome is 1.7 (95% CI 1.2–2.6).
- Patients treated with TPA are 30–50% more likely (relative risk increase) to have minimal or no disability at 3 months.
- NNT (number needed to treat) = 3 to result in 1 patient with better outcome than if not treated.
- NNH (number needed to harm) = 33 to result in 1 patient with worse outcome than if not treated.

WHO BENEFITS?

Subgroups:
- All stroke subtypes benefit.
- Both mild (NIHSS ≤ 7) and severe (NIHSS ≥ 15) stroke patients benefit.
- Elderly (>75 years) as well as young patients benefit, but there are little data in the pediatric population.
- Patients with early ischemic changes on CT still benefit if they meet all other criteria.
- Time to treatment is the key to an improved chance of recovery.[15] Patients treated earlier are more likely to respond than those treated at the end of the 3-hour time window. Therefore, **time is brain!**

WHO IS MORE LIKELY TO BLEED?

- Patients with more severe stroke.
- Patients with extensive CT changes, elevated BP, glucose, and temperature, and those of advanced age.
- But **even those with severe strokes, early CT changes, and advanced age show overall benefit with TPA treatment**, even accounting for the chances of bleeding. This is because, without treatment, such patients are universally going to do poorly.[16,17]

■ Unproven therapies

INTRA-ARTERIAL (IA) THERAPY WITHIN 3 HOURS

Within the 3-hour time window, only IV TPA is approved. There still has been no direct comparison of IA therapy vs. IV TPA within 3 hours of symptom onset.

Therefore, if a patient qualifies within 3 hours for IV TPA, but, because of persisting arterial occlusion you think the patient might also benefit from IA therapy, **do not withhold IV TPA in favor of IA therapy**. The Interventional Management of Stroke (IMS) I, II, and III trials are ongoing in North America to determine if IA treatment following IV TPA is beneficial compared to just IV TPA. If you choose to proceed to IA, still treat with IV conventional dose first. Generally, in these IA cases, we are using more mechanical methods rather than more lytic drugs to get the artery open.

There are several reasons for this recommendation, but mainly we do not want to deprive someone of proven effective IV TPA in favor of something (IA therapy) that remains unproven. Also, we have found that when we decide to go directly to IA, some patients may never get treated, or their treatment will be delayed, for logistical reasons (mobilizing the angiography team, equipment failure, difficulty with catheterization, etc.). In 10–20% of those we treated with IV TPA first and then took for IA treatment, we found that the clot was already lysed by the IV drug by the time we got the artery catheterized, so that had we not given IV TPA, lysis would not have occurred as soon. Finally, the IMS study experience of IV followed by IA therapy has shown that this approach is no more risky than either IV TPA or IA alone.[18]

INTRAVENOUS LYTICS OR INTRA-ARTERIAL THERAPY BEYOND 3 HOURS

Beyond 3 hours, both IV and IA approaches are being evaluated, based on pooled data from all patients treated with IV TPA, showing that there may be some benefit at least to 5 hours after symptom onset.[19] Furthermore, physiologic brain imaging purports to demonstrate reversibly damaged penumbral tissue for up to 12–24 hours in some cases. However, such therapy is **not approved** by the FDA in the USA, or by other regulatory agencies in other countries. This is because the clinical efficacy of treatment beyond 3 hours has never been proven in a prospective randomized trial. At some time point after symptom onset in most stroke patients, it may be worse to open an artery than to leave it occluded, if the tissue is already dead and non-salvageable, since such tissue is at increased risk of bleeding during reperfusion.

Several studies of either IV or IA treatment up to 9 hours after symptom onset are ongoing based on the assumption that there is a subset of patients who can still safely respond to treatment in the 3–9-hour interval. Most of these studies are using CT and MRI to identify those patients who have persisting occlusion, who still harbor salvageable tissue, and in whom the existing damage is not so severe that recanalization would be excessively risky. This rapidly moving area of stroke research should be clarified by the completion of these trials in the next year or so. Unfortunately, none of these studies are directly comparing IV to IA treatment, and existing case series do not demonstrate a clear superiority in terms of either safety or clinical outcome of either approach beyond 3 hours.

IA therapy refers to IA thrombolytics given directly into the clot, mechanical clot disruption, or both. In general, the trend is toward more mechanical methods, particularly in those patients who have already received IV TPA, or who have contraindications (for instance, elevated INR) to thrombolytics. The MERCI retrieval catheter and device has been approved by the FDA to open cerebral arterial occlusions, but has not yet been shown to improve outcome compared to standard treatment.[20]

WHO SHOULD BE CONSIDERED FOR IA THERAPY?

- Patients who have received IV TPA for a distal ICA, M1 segment of MCA, proximal M2 segment of MCA, or basilar lesion on TCD, MRA, or CTA, who have not recanalized by the time they get to the angio suite, and who still have a disabling deficit. Even if patients have received full-dose IV TPA, we have found that following IV therapy with IA therapy is safe in most patients. However, this must still be done while the tissue is still alive, i.e., before there are extensive ischemic CT changes or while the MRI still shows mismatch (see Appendix 5).

- Patients who qualify for IV TPA within 3 hours but have certain exclusions that would increase bleeding risk, such as recent major surgery or INR > 1.6, and who have a devastating stroke. However, IA thrombolysis has been associated with up to 10% rates of symptomatic ICH, so IA lytics should not be considered a "safer" alternative to IV TPA. But IA therapy allows the use of mechanical clot disruption rather than pharmacologic clot lysis, and these mechanical approaches might be associated with less bleeding risk in such patients.

- Patients outside the 3-hour window but within 9 hours of onset of symptoms, with a severe stroke (NIHSS ≥ 10), limited or no ischemic changes on CT, significant perfusion/diffusion mismatch on MRI (see Appendix 5), with no other contraindication. In these cases, we consider either IV TPA or IA therapy depending on whether we can identify a large artery occlusion on TCD, MRA, or CTA, and the availability of the endovascular team to mobilize quickly. We often push the time window for starting IA therapy beyond 9 hours if the patient has a suspected basilar occlusion, because doing nothing would be uniformly fatal.

5

Neurological deterioration in acute ischemic stroke

Although classically stroke symptoms are maximal at onset and patients gradually recover over days, weeks, and months, patients can deteriorate. People have termed the phenomenon stroke progression, stroke in evolution, stroke deterioration, and symptom fluctuation. There is no consistent terminology. The phenomenon occurs from different causes and is incompletely understood. This chapter will discuss evaluation of potential causes, and approaches for treatment of each cause.

■ Probable causes

(1) Stroke enlargement (e.g., arterial stenosis or occlusion with worsening perfusion).
(2) Drop in perfusion pressure.
(3) Recurrent stroke (not common).
(4) Cerebral edema and mass effect.
(5) Hemorrhagic transformation.
(6) Metabolic disturbance (decreased O_2 saturation, decreased cardiac output, increased glucose, decreased sodium, fever, sedative drugs, etc.).
(7) Seizure, post-ictal.

(8) Symptom fluctuation without good cause (due to inflammation?).

(9) The patient is not feeling like cooperating (sleepy, drugs).

■ Initial evaluation of patients with neurologic deterioration

- Check airway–breathing–circulation, vital signs, laboratory tests. Is the patient hypotensive or hypoxic?
- Talk to and examine the patient. If the patient is sleepy, is it because it's 3 a.m. or because of mass effect? Is there a pattern of symptoms (global worsening vs. focal worsening)?
- Get an immediate non-contrast head CT (to evaluate for hemorrhage, new stroke, swelling, etc.).
- Review medications (antihypertensives, sedatives).
- Observe patient, and ask nurse, for subtle signs of seizure.
- Consider MRI for arterial imaging, new stroke, stroke enlargement, swelling; TCD or CT angiography for arterial imaging; EEG to diagnose subclinical seizures.

■ Stroke enlargement

This occurs when there is arterial stenosis or occlusion and the hemodynamics change for whatever reason. There are no data to support that anticoagulation prevents the hemodynamic worsening, though many clinicians jump to anticoagulation with heparin. Instead, probably the best treatment is to treat the underlying stenosis/occlusion early.

The approach should be to prevent rather than treat after deterioration. The key is early imaging to detect large artery stenosis/occlusion by TCD, CT angiography, or MRI (i.e., find the high-risk patients early). Patients with minor deficits but abnormal TCD or MRA are at highest risk of progression. Perfusion imaging may indicate areas of tissue at risk. Even without a perfusion study by MRI or CT, the finding of a small diffusion-weighted lesion on MRI and a relatively minor neurological deficit in the presence of large artery occlusion by arterial imaging indicates a high risk for progression.

In such patients, you might want to consider early intervention, such as IV thrombolysis despite low NIHSS score, intra-arterial therapy, carotid endarterectomy, or carotid stenting.

■ Drop in perfusion pressure

Since autoregulation is lost in ischemic brain, any reduction in blood pressure will reduce flow to penumbral regions, thereby potentially worsening the clinical deficit. This is true in both cortical and subcortical strokes. The latter have particularly poor collateral flow and may be at greatest risk for hypoperfusion-related deterioration. As a rule of thumb, mean arterial pressure (MAP) should be kept at pre-stroke levels (as a general guideline, at least 130 mm Hg in hypertensive patients, and 110 in normotensive patients) in the first 24 hours, and if MAP drops below this level, and the patient deteriorates, the MAP should be increased by a fluid bolus and possibly a pressor. Don't forget head positioning. Simply laying the patient flat, or no higher than 15° head elevation, may augment cerebral perfusion.

■ Recurrent stroke

Unfortunately some patients go on to have recurrent stroke. Among atrial fibrillation patients, the stroke recurrence risk has been reported to be 5–8% in the first two weeks.[5,6,21*] There are no data to show that immediate or "early" anticoagulation helps, even in the setting of atrial fibrillation, because anticoagulation can lead to hemorrhagic complications (see **Hemorrhagic transformation**, below).

Yet we might be underestimating the magnitude of frequency of stroke recurrence if we rely on clinical deterioration alone. One study reported stroke recurrence was detected by MRI in 34% of patients in the first week, whereas clinically only 2% stroke recurrence was noted.[22] Furthermore, some patients may be at higher risk of re-embolization, especially those with associated mitral stenosis or left atrial thrombus. Therefore, our recommendation in atrial fibrillation patients is to anticoagulate once we determine by repeat brain imaging that the infarct is small or, if large, that any acute hemorrhagic transformation or vasogenic edema is resolving. This usually means waiting 48–96 hours after the acute stroke.

In a larger population-based study, large artery atherosclerosis was associated with highest risk of stroke recurrence (Table 5.1 and Fig. 5.1).[23] This supports the recommendation to perform carotid revascularization (endarterectomy or stenting) earlier than later (See **Carotid stenosis**, Chapter 6).

■ Cerebral edema and mass effect

This is a worry with large strokes, such as big MCA strokes involving the basal ganglia, often with some involvement of the ACA or PCA territories as well, and large cerebellar strokes. It is a worry with young patients who do not have much atrophy and thus not much room for the brain to swell inside the skull.

Monitor for any neurologic change, decline in level of consciousness, rising blood pressure, periodic breathing, hiccups,

Table 5.1. Stroke mechanisms and risk of early recurrence.

Mechanism	Recurrence at 1 week (95% CI)	Recurrence at 1 month (95% CI)	Recurrence at 3 months (95% CI)
Large artery atherosclerosis (LAA)	4.0% (0.2–7.8)	12.6% (5.9–19.3)	19.2% (11.2–27.2)
Cardioembolism (CE)	2.5% (0.1–4.9)	4.6% (1.3–7.9)	11.9% (6.4–17.4)
Small-vessel stroke (SVS)	0%	2.0% (0–4.2)	3.4% (0.5–6.3)
Undetermined (UND)	2.3% (0.5–4.1)	6.5% (3.4–9.6)	9.3% (5.6–13.0)

Adapted from: J. K. Lovett, A. J. Coull, & P. M. Rothwell, Early risk of recurrence by subtype of ischemic stroke in population-based incidence studies. *Neurology* 2004; **62**: 569–73.[23] Reproduced with permission from Lippincott Williams & Wilkins.

headache, new cranial nerve abnormalities, and pupils (late phenomenon).

MEDICAL TREATMENT

- Most important is good post-stroke care such as head positioning ($\leq 15°$), immediate correction of fever, electrolyte imbalance, and hyperglycemia, and careful optimization of MAP and cardiac output to insure adequate cerebral perfusion.
- Do not give steroids* (grade A recommendation). Randomized studies have shown that steroids may be harmful rather than beneficial after acute stroke.
- Osmotherapy (i.e., mannitol) is a temporizing measure that may help in some cases. Give mannitol (0.5–1 g/kg bolus over

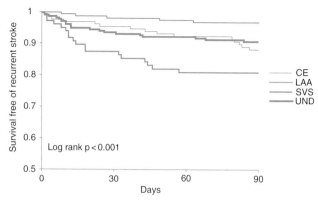

Figure 5.1. Stroke recurrence risk by stroke mechanism.[23]
Note: See Table 5.1 for abbreviations.
Adapted from: J. K. Lovett, A. J. Coull, & P. M. Rothwell, Early risk of recurrence by subtype of ischemic stroke in population-based incidence studies. *Neurology* 2004; **62**: 569–73.[23] Reproduced with permission from Lippincott Williams & Wilkins.

30–60 minutes, and then 0.25 g/kg every 6 hours) aiming to increase baseline serum osmolality by 10%, but no higher than 315 mosm. Check serum osmolality every 12 hours and hold mannitol if >315 mosm.
- Cerebrospinal fluid drainage by ventriculostomy may help if hydrocephalus is contributing to increase ICP.

SURGICAL THERAPY

- Obtain neurosurgical consultation early.
- For large MCA infarcts, consider early decompressive hemi-craniectomy. The skull is taken off (and put in freezer) and dural incision is made so that the brain can swell out rather than compress the brainstem (see below).

- For cerebellar stroke, the appropriate treatment is posterior fossa decompression and cerebellectomy.
- With both procedures, a common error is not to remove enough bone, resulting in inadequate decompression. Be sure the neurosurgeon knows the anatomical guidelines for decompression. They are included below as a guide and Fig. 5.2 shows an outline of the surgical method.

Decompressive surgery is a life-saving measure. While it has never been proven effective in a randomized study, most stroke experts recommend it in highly selected cases based on case series. It is particularly recommended for large cerebellar strokes, as people can be quite functional without a large part of their cerebellum. However, with respect to large MCA strokes, talk with family about quality of life after stroke survival versus death. Many do not perform the procedure as often for large left MCA strokes as the patient is likely to be left aphasic. Age is an important predictor of outcome after hemicraniectomy, all other things being equal, with less likelihood of acceptable outcome in patients over 60 years old. Best results occur with early intervention in young patients with non-dominant-hemisphere strokes.

Criteria for consideration of hemicraniectomy
- <5 hrs from onset; >50% MCA territory hypodense
- <48 hrs from onset; complete MCA territory hypodense
- >7.5 mm midline shift
- >4 mm midline shift with lethargy

Other criteria include:
- age < 60
- 145 cc infarct volume on MRI

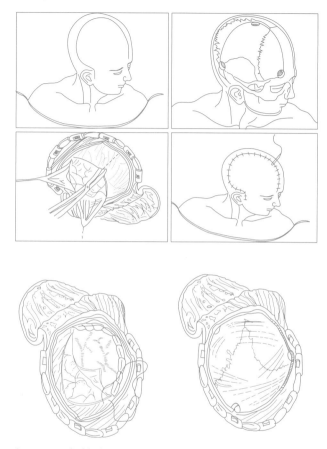

Figure 5.2. Method for hemicraniectomy.

Guidelines for adequate surgical decompression from ongoing clinical trials

- anterior: frontal to mid-pupillary line
- posterior: 4 cm posterior to external auditory canal

- superior: superior sagittal sinus
- inferior: floor of middle cranial fossa
- durotomy over the entire region of decompression
- dural grafting

Other criteria include:

  - 12 cm diameter craniectomy

■ Hemorrhagic transformation

This should be clearly visible on non-contrast head CT
(Fig. 5.3). Most of the time, the patient is asymptomatic from
the hemorrhagic transformation (also known as hemorrhagic
conversion), unless it is large or in a critical location.
Radiographically, hemorrhagic transformation is divided into
four categories.[24]

- Hemorrhagic infarct 1 and 2 (HI1 and HI2) represent pete-
  chial bleeding into the area of infarct without mass effect and
  are rarely symptomatic. HI1 are small petechiae. HI2 are
  confluent.

If HI occurs, usually there is not much you can do or should do,
except to stop antiplatelets and anticoagulants temporarily
until you are sure there is no continued bleeding on repeat
brain imaging.

- Parenchymal hemorrhage 1 and 2 (PH1 and PH2) represent
  confluent bleeding. If the bleeding takes up more than 30% of
  the infarcted area and produces mass effect (PH2), it usually
  produces neurological deterioration.

The risk of developing PH2 is the main reason why anticoagulation is not recommended immediately after cardioembolic
stroke, and without repeat brain imaging first. These should
be managed similarly to any other cerebral hemorrhage
(Chapter 8).

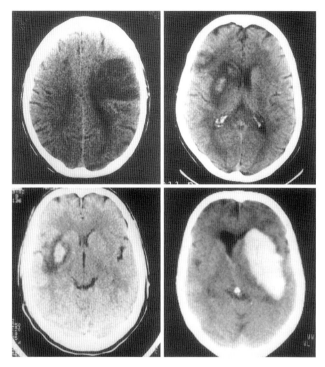

Figure 5.3. Types of hemorrhagic transformation: HI1 (top left), HI2 (top right), PH1 (bottom left), and PH2 (bottom right).[24]

Source: M. Fiorelli, S. Bastianello, R. von Kummer, *et al.*, Hemorrhagic transformation within 36 hours of a cerebral infarct: relationships with early clinical deterioration and 3-month outcome in the European Cooperative Acute Stroke Study I (ECASS I) cohort. *Stroke* 1999; **30**: 2280–4.[24] Reproduced with permission from Lippincott Williams & Wilkins.

■ Metabolic disturbance

These are pretty self-explanatory. Remember that a sick brain is more sensitive to the effects of metabolic perturbations, so these should be sought and aggressively treated.

- Mild fever or changes in sodium or glucose may have an exaggerated clinical effect.
- Any intercurrent infection such as urinary tract infection or pneumonia will magnify the neurologic findings.
- Reduced cardiac output is a particularly bad comorbidity resulting in worse clinical outcome, and should be carefully avoided by optimizing fluid and inotropic therapy.
- Remember also that "if the lips are blue, the brain is too," so look for, determine the cause of, and treat arterial oxygen desaturation. Possible causes:
  - pulmonary embolism
  - pneumonia
  - pulmonary edema
- Anemia: transfuse for hemoglobin < 10 g.
- Sedative drugs interfere with rapid transition to rehabilitation mode and have also been associated with worse outcome, decreased mobilization with attendant increased DVT, etc. Sedating drugs should be avoided as far as possible. See **The uncooperative patient**, below.

■ Seizure

Seizures occur in roughly 20% of all strokes, and are somewhat more frequent after hemorrhage than infarct. Most of the time, if seizures occur, they will appear at the time of stroke onset or within 24 hours. Seizures will often cause a post-ictal depressed level of consciousness, as well as worsening of the focal signs.

- Most authorities recommend withholding anticonvulsants unless the seizures are recurrent.
- Status epilepticus after acute stroke is exceedingly rare.
- For recurrent seizures or status, start with fosphenytoin 20 mg/kg IV, then after 12 hours maintenance phenytoin 200–300 mg per day.
- Intubation may be necessary to protect the airway in patients who already are impaired from their stroke.
- Aspiration pneumonia is common after seizures and should be assumed to occur if the seizure is generalized or intubation is necessary.
- If delayed or recurrent seizures occur, then non-sedating anticonvulsants such as the following are recommended, in this order:
  - lamotrigine: 25 mg per day titrating up every 2 weeks by 50 mg to 150 mg per day
  - gabapentin: 300 mg per day titrating up every 3–4 days to 1500 mg per day in divided doses
  - levetiracetam: 500 mg every 12 hours titrating up every 2 weeks to 2000 mg per day

■ Symptom fluctuations without a good cause

Some patients deteriorate without an obvious explanation. This is a poorly understood phenomenon. It is commonly seen with subcortical strokes. While this usually occurs in the first three days, it can occur up to two weeks after stroke onset.

The mechanism is unknown. Local hypoperfusion? Inflammation? Neurochemical or neurotransmitter changes? Apoptosis?

Treatment is mainly supportive (maintain euvolemia, check blood pressure to make sure it doesn't drop, put head of bed flat). Anti-inflammatory (i.e., high-dose statins) and other neuroprotective therapies are under evaluation. One recent study of a free radical trapping drug showed improved outcome in acute ischemic stroke patients, indirectly supporting the laboratory evidence demonstrating an important role of inflammation in producing damage after stroke.[25]

■ The uncooperative patient

Patients can become confused after a stroke. Contributing factors include advanced age and underlying dementia, placement in a disorienting critical-care environment, and sleep deprivation. Often, movement to a quiet private room helps, but this has to be balanced against less close scrutiny and treatment of medical complications outside the stroke unit or ICU setting. While sedation should be avoided, low doses of antipsychotic agents can be useful and are used commonly – such as haloperidol PO or IV 0.5–2.0 mg, risperidone 1 mg PO and quetiapine 25 mg PO. There are also data to suggest that newer antipsychotic agents increase mortality of patients with dementia, though this was with prolonged treatment (10–12 weeks).[26] Therefore pharmacologic management of agitation and confusion should be practiced with caution. Good nursing care, orientation, and calm environment are important.

6

Ischemic stroke prevention: why we do the things we do

In this chapter, we discuss mainly secondary prevention for stroke, although many of the measures, especially control of risk factors and lifestyle changes such as not smoking, controlling blood pressure, etc., are also important measures to avoid a first stroke.

Initially, we discuss a tailored diagnostic work-up, then general measures for secondary prevention of ischemic stroke, and finally recommendations for specific conditions that are associated with a high risk of stroke.

■ Investigations

The goal of the "stroke work-up" is to find the cause of the stroke in order to determine the best treatment options to maximize the chance of preventing another stroke.

A thorough ischemic stroke work-up is not just CT/MRI/MRA/ECHO/CAROTIDS/TCD/LIPIDS/HBA1C.

There is no "cookbook" work-up for ischemic stroke. It is important to consider the patient's risk factors and stroke syndrome when determining the extent of the diagnostic evaluation. For instance, a 75-year-old man with longstanding hypertension, diabetes, and hypercholesterolemia and a lacunar infarct confirmed on brain imaging may need little additional work-up beyond a carotid ultrasound and EKG. However, a 40-year-old man with no known risk factors and an acute stroke would require an extensive evaluation.

The following is a list of the studies that we **consider** in most stroke patients to distinguish stroke subtype and tailor our preventive measures. In Appendix 12 we will address the additional evaluation for young stroke patients with no risk factors, and others where the underlying cause may be more obscure. In addition to the following, almost all stroke patients should have a complete blood count, electrolytes, creatinine, blood glucose, INR, PTT, and electrocardiogram (see standard orders in Appendix 3).

Initial acute head CT[*]

- To rule out ICH and other causes, to assess for old strokes, to detect early signs of ischemia.

MRI of the brain/MRA of the neck and brain (circle of Willis)

- To localize the lesion.
- To try to understand the mechanism by integrating all MRI and MRA data:
  - small-vessel lacunar infarction
  - large-artery atherosclerosis
  - embolism
  - hemodynamic
  - venous
- To say what's acute and what's old using diffusion-weighted sequence.
- To understand the tissue physiology (perfusion imaging).

- To examine the entire cervical and cerebral vasculature for stenosis (atherosclerosis, dissection, etc.), aneurysm, arteriovenous malformation (AVM).
- You can see many unexpected things, including incidental findings.

Possibly, repeat head CT

- To localize the lesion, if patient is unable to have an MRI.
- To evaluate the deteriorating patient:
  - to assess mass effect/edema
  - to look for hemorrhagic conversion
  - to look for stroke recurrence

CT angiogram (CTA) of the neck and brain (circle of Willis)

- To look for arterial stenosis, dissection, aneurysm (especially if the patient is unable to have an MRI).

Transthoracic echocardiogram (TTE) (order with "bubble study")

- To assess for embolic source (anterior wall or apical akinesis, clot, valvular disease, large PFO).
- Low ejection fraction (20–30% is generally agreed upon as a cutoff) significantly increases thromboembolic risk due to stasis, and also should trigger further specific cardiac evaluation and treatment.

Transesophageal echocardiogram (TEE) (order with "bubble study")

- To assess for embolic source not seen well on TTE (aortic atheroma, PFO, atrial septal aneurysm, spontaneous echo contrast, left atrial appendage clot).

- If a PFO is found, we often will also do a screen for hyper-coagulable states, a bilateral lower extremity ultrasound, and MR venogram of the pelvis to look for venous thrombosis. See discussion on PFO at the end of this chapter.

Carotid ultrasound (CUS)
- To assess for internal carotid artery stenosis or occlusion.
- Shows you direction of vertebral artery flow.
- You might not need it if you have a good-quality normal MRA or CTA of the extracranial circulation. CUS can be used to confirm a stenosis seen on MRA or CTA. If these non-invasive tests are concordant, it may not be necessary to do an invasive DSA to determine candidacy for endovascular or surgical treatment of a carotid stenosis.

Transcranial Doppler (with or without bubble study)
- To monitor clot presence and lysis in the acute setting.
- To confirm intracranial stenosis/occlusion of major arteries seen on MRA or CTA.
- Emboli detection/monitoring.
- Look for PFO by injecting microbubbles. TCD with "bubble study" is the most sensitive and least expensive/invasive way to screen for right to left shunting.
- Hemodynamic reserve (breath holding index, vasomotor reactivity).
- Evaluate collateral flow patterns.

Digital subtraction angiography (DSA)
- Gold standard for determining degree of stenosis.
- Only way to definitively delineate and follow aneurysms or AVMs, dissection, vasculitis, or other arteriopathies.

Fasting lipids

- Look for high total cholesterol, triglycerides, LDL (target LDL < 100 mg/dL; for very high-risk patients LDL < 70 mg/dL).
- Look for low HDL.

Hemoglobin A1c (HbA1c)

- Screen for diabetes and its recent control.

■ Ischemic stroke prevention: general measures

Educate your patients so they can take an active role in their health care and secondary prevention of ischemic stroke.

Try to convert patients to the medications that they will be going home on prior to discharge, to make sure they tolerate them. Also, take cost issues into account. A patient who cannot afford the medications will not take them.

The following are derived from the most recently published guidelines, which should be consulted for details.[27]

(1) CONTROL RISK FACTORS

- Hypertension(based on SHEP trial, and others).[28*] See below for more detail.
  - ACE inhibitors (HOPE, PROGRESS trials).[29,30*]
  - Diuretics and calcium channel blockers (ALLHAT trial).[31*]
- Elevated lipids:
  - Statins (several trials, including MRC Heart Protection Study).[32]
  - Target LDL ≤ 70 mg/dl according to the most recent guidelines for high-risk cardiovascular patients.[33]

- Be sure to get baseline liver functions before starting statin therapy.
- Smoking:
  - Cessation counseling and pharmacotherapy.
- Diabetes:
  - Identification.
  - Treatment, including diet.
- Hyperhomocysteinemia:
  - May justify folic acid, B12, B6 treatment, but so far there is no evidence that vitamins – including folic acid – are effective for stroke prevention in general (VISP study).[34]
  - Therefore, since there is no effective treatment for this risk factor for stroke, routine screening for hyperhomocysteinemia is probably not cost-effective.
- Estrogen use (WEST trial, Women's Health Initiative):[35–37*]
  - Avoid in most cases.
- Drugs of abuse and alcohol:
  - Should be avoided and discouraged, especially vasoactive drugs such as cocaine and amphetamines.
  - No more than two drinks per day.

(2) ANTITHROMBOTIC OR ANTICOAGULANT MEDICATIONS

- Aspirin (many studies).[38*] ~20% relative risk reduction of secondary stroke/other vascular events. Doses of 50 mg daily or higher; usually give 81 or 325 mg.
- Aspirin/dipyridamole ER (Aggrenox, Asasantin). ESPS-1 and ESPS-2 trials; 30% better than aspirin alone.[39,40*]
  - The PRoFESS trial (ongoing) is comparing aspirin/dipyridamole ER (Aggrenox) to clopidogrel (Plavix).

- Clopidogrel (Plavix). CAPRIE trial.[41*] Slightly better than aspirin, particularly in patients with peripheral vascular disease, and better tolerated.
- Aspirin/clopidogrel combination. Long-term use increases bleeding rate without benefit of greater stroke prevention (MATCH and CHARISMA studies).[42,43] Therefore the combination is not recommended long-term (more than a few days) unless the patient has had a recent stent placed.
- Warfarin (Coumadin). For most of the following, the use of warfarin can be considered based on either randomized trials (level A) or consensus recommendations (level C). However, except for those with Class 1 evidence (i.e., where there is general agreement with its use), either antiplatelet drugs or warfarin can be used.
  - Atrial fibrillation except for "lone AF" (see below) (SPAF trials).[44,45*] Class 1, level A evidence.
  - Critical extracranial carotid stenosis. String sign or occlusion (anecdotal experience).
  - Basilar thrombosis/stenosis (anecdotal experience).
  - Arterial dissection (consensus statements).
  - Other "embologenic" cardiac conditions:[46]
    - rheumatic valvular disease or mechanical valve (class 1 evidence)
    - low left ventricular ejection fraction (<30%) (consensus statements)
    - akinesis or severe hypokinesis of left ventricle segments (especially anterior wall or apex) (consensus statements)
    - stroke soon after myocardial infarction, especially if mural thrombus is identified on TTE (randomized studies)

- aortic atheroma > 4 mm (from SPAF III subgroup analysis, consensus recommendation)[47,48]
- Embolic-looking cryptogenic stroke (randomized trial – WARSS subgroup analysis)[49,50]
- Stroke patients with documented coagulopathy (consensus statements)
  - Especially if history or evidence of venous thrombosis, or pulmonary embolism
  - Also patients with full antiphospholipid antibody syndrome (venous thrombosis, miscarriages, livedo reticularis)
- Venous infarction due to cerebral venous sinus thrombosis (consensus statements)
- Based on the following randomized trials, warfarin is **not** routinely indicated for:
  - stroke due to intracranial atherosclerosis (WASID study),[51]
  - most non-cardioembolic strokes (WARSS),[52]
  - most stroke patients with positive antiphospholipid antibody (APASS: a WARSS substudy),[53] or
  - most patients with PFO (PICCS: a WARSS substudy).[50*]

(3) LIFESTYLE MODIFICATION

Lifestyle modification may reduce the risk factors mentioned above.

- Stop smoking. This is one of the most important things patients can do, to prevent not only ischemic stroke but also heart disease, lung cancer, and head and neck cancer, etc.
- Better diet. Refer patients to a dietician who can talk with patients about a low-fat diet and diabetic diet if applicable.
- More exercise. Counsel the patient to adopt a less sedentary lifestyle and participate in even moderate exercise.

(4) BLOOD PRESSURE CONTROL*

Hypertension is the single most important modifiable risk factor. JNC 7 reports that the risk of cardiovascular disease, beginning at 115/75 mm Hg, doubles with each increment of 20/10 mm Hg.[54]

- Multiple large randomized controlled trials have shown efficacy of antihypertensive treatment in primary and secondary prevention of stroke. The selection of antihypertensives remains unsettled and controversial.
- Many drugs have been shown to reduce stroke in primary prevention (beta-blocker in SHEP, diuretic in SHEP and ALLHAT, calcium channel blocker in ALLHAT, ACE inhibitor in HOPE and PROGRESS, ARB in LIFE).[28–31,55]
- A combination of perindopril (Aceon), a tissue-specific ACE inhibitor, and indapamide (Lozol), a diuretic, have been shown to reduce stroke in secondary prevention even among non-hypertensive patients (PROGRESS).[30] Whether this effect is due to the tissue-specific ACE inhibition rather than an ACE-inhibitor class effect, or whether an ACE inhibitor needs to be used in combination with a diuretic, remains controversial.
- Probably the most important point is blood pressure reduction, not the specific drug. For primary prevention, a diuretic seems to be effective and cheap. Recent meta-analysis seems to support the superiority of diuretics.[56] JNC 7 also recommends thiazide diuretics as a first-line pharmacologic therapy, though it recognizes that more than one drug is commonly needed.
- In the hospital setting, especially after a stroke, a patient's fluid intake may be poor. A diuretic while on IV fluids does not make sense. **Start a diuretic in stroke inpatients only if the patient is drinking fluids consistently**.

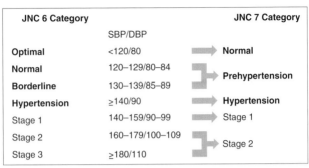

JNC 6 Category	SBP/DBP	JNC 7 Category
Optimal	<120/80	**Normal**
Normal	120–129/80–84	**Prehypertension**
Borderline	130–139/85–89	
Hypertension	≥140/90	**Hypertension**
Stage 1	140–159/90–99	Stage 1
Stage 2	160–179/100–109	Stage 2
Stage 3	≥180/110	

Sources: The sixth report of the Joint National Committee on Prevention, Detection, Evaluation, and Treatment of High Blood Pressure. *Arch Intern Med* 1997;**157**:2413–46.
The seventh report of the Joint National Committee on Prevention, Detection, Evaluation, and Treatment of High Blood Pressure. *JAMA* 2003;**289**:2560–2571.

Figure 6.1. Recent JNC 6 and 7 blood pressure categories.[54]

- **Bring down BP slowly** with oral antihypertensives after acute ischemic stroke.
- According to recent guidelines (Fig. 6.1), the **target blood pressures** are the following:
  - <140/90 mm Hg
  - <130/80 mm Hg for patients with diabetes or chronic kidney disease
- Remember, there is a continuous increase in risk of stroke with increase in blood pressure. There is no biological cutoff point.

■ Atrial fibrillation (A fib)

A great deal is known about the prevention of stroke due to atrial fibrillation, and effective treatment is available. For a good review see Hart *et al.*, 2003.[44]

IN THE ACUTE STROKE SETTING

- Acute stroke recurrence rate estimates vary.
- From International Stroke Trial: 3.9% stroke recurrence rate in 14 days.[21]
- Therefore, there is no reason to rush to anticoagulate with heparin or warfarin after an A-fib-related stroke. Wait 48–96 hours after a major stroke and repeat the CT (or MRI) first to exclude hemorrhagic transformation.

NATURAL HISTORY OF CHRONIC ATRIAL FIBRILLATION

- Valvular atrial fibrillation: stroke risk ~17 × that of controls.
- Non-valvular atrial fibrillation: stroke risk 6 × controls or ~5% per year.
- Risk stratification:
  - Low risk: "lone" atrial fibrillation: age < 60, none of the risk factors listed below, and no history of TIA, stroke, or other embolic event: 0.5% stroke risk per year.
  - Moderate and high risk: variable combinations of age > 75, decreased left ventricular function, hypertension, diabetes, and previous cardioembolism: up to 10% stroke risk per year.
  - Prior stroke/TIA/embolism: >10% stroke risk per year.
  - **So, by definition, any atrial-fibrillation patient with embolic stroke or TIA is considered "high risk."**
  - Age > 80: >7% per year.
  - Echocardiographic risk features include: left ventricular dysfunction, left atrial enlargement or clot, mitral annular calcification, spontaneous echo contrast.

TREATMENT OF CHRONIC ATRIAL FIBRILLATION

- The choice of antiplatelet therapy vs. warfarin depends on the risk of stroke. Table 6.1 shows the risk reduction with treatment of A-fib patients according to their various risk categories.

Primary stroke prevention with warfarin (Coumadin)*

- Ischemic stroke risk decreased to ~2% per year, or ~60% relative risk reduction.
- Major bleeding risk: 1.5%–2% per year.
  - Increased risk with recent hemorrhage, falling, advanced age, alcohol binge, closed head injury, liver disease, aspirin, NSAIDs, cancer, age, previous stroke, uncontrolled hypertension.
- ICH risk: 0.2–0.4% per year.
  - Age ≤ 75: 0.5% per year (data from SPAFII).
  - Age > 75: 1.8% per year.
- Target therapeutic INR is 2.0–3.0.

Primary stroke prevention with aspirin*

- Ischemic stroke risk decreased to ~4% per year, or 20% relative risk reduction.
- Major bleeding risk: 0.3–0.9 % per year.
- ICH risk: 0–0.3% per year.

SECONDARY PREVENTION (MOST OF OUR CASES ON THE STROKE SERVICE)

- Warfarin reduces the risk of recurrent ischemic stroke from 10–12% per year to 4% per year.*
- Target INR: 2.0–3.0.

Table 6.1. Stroke risk reduction with aspirin and warfarin in different groups of patients with atrial fibrillation.

Risk strata	Stroke rate with aspirin (%/y)	Relative risk reduction: warfarin vs. aspirin (%)[a]	NNT$_B$[b]	General recommendation
Previous stroke or transient ischemic attack	10	60	17	Warfarin (INR 2–3)
Primary prevention				
High risk	>4	55	35	Warfarin (INR 2–3)
Moderate risk	2–4	45	75	Warfarin or aspirin[c]
Low risk	<2	35	>200	Aspirin (81–235 mg/d)

Notes:

Step 1: Estimate the patient's risk for stroke given aspirin. Several clinical schemes to stratify stroke risk in atrial fibrillation have been published; the Stroke Prevention in Atrial Fibrillation III scheme has been most widely validated.

Step 2: Identify any special risks for hemorrhage during anticoagulation.

Step 3: Based on estimated stroke risk and contraindications for anticoagulation, consider use of warfarin or aspirin.

INR = international normalized ratio

NNT$_B$ = number needed to treat for benefit

[a] The best overall estimate of relative risk reduction in stroke by warfarin over aspirin in unselected patients with atrial fibrillation is about 45%, but the magnitude varies with the inherent rate of stroke because of the varying ratios of warfarin-sensitive cardioembolic strokes to warfarin-insensitive noncardioembolic strokes.

Notes to Table 6.1. (cont.)

[b] NNT$_B$ for 1 year with warfarin instead of aspirin to prevent one stroke, calculated on the basis of stroke rates of 10%, 5%, 3%, and 1% per year on aspirin for previous stroke, high-risk primary prevention, moderate risk, and low risk, respectively.

[c] The choice of warfarin vs. aspirin should particularly consider patient values or preferences, individual bleeding risk, and availability of reliable anticoagulation monitoring.

Adapted from: R. G. Hart, J. L. Halperin, L. A. Pearce, *et al.*, Lessons from the Stroke Prevention in Atrial Fibrillation trials. *Ann. Intern. Med.* 2003; **138**: 831–8.[44] Reproduced with permission from the American College of Physicians.

■ Carotid stenosis

Carotid stenosis is also one of the better-studied causes of stroke for which specific therapy is available. There is a large body of literature on carotid endarterectomy and a large one is developing for carotid stenting. For review we recommend Barnett *et al.*, 2002.[57]

SYMPTOMATIC INTERNAL CAROTID STENOSIS (70–99% BY NASCET CRITERIA OF ANGIOGRAPHIC STENOSIS)

- Surgery (carotid endarterectomy, CEA) is beneficial compared to medical therapy.[58*]
  - 2-year risk of ipsilateral stroke was 8.6% in the surgical group and 24.5% in the medical group (RRR 65%, ARR 16%, NNT 6 to prevent 1 stroke in 2 years).
  - It is most beneficial to those who have highest risk of subsequent stroke: those who had hemispheric symptoms (compared to ocular symptoms), tandem extracranial and

intracranial disease, and those without apparent collaterals.

■ Perioperative risk was 5.8% overall and was higher for those with contralateral internal carotid occlusion and those with intraluminal thrombus, but those high-risk patients still received benefit.

SYMPTOMATIC STENOSIS (50–69%)

• Benefit of surgery is marginal.
  ■ 5-year risk of any ipsilateral stroke was 15.7% surgical vs. 22.2% medical (ARR 7%, $p = 0.045$).*
  ■ No benefit in preventing disabling strokes.
  ■ Women and those whose symptoms were limited to transient monocular blindness did not benefit.
  ■ 6.7% 1-month surgical morbidity and mortality in NASCET.

ASYMPTOMATIC STENOSIS

• The risks vs. benefits of treating asymptomatic carotid stenosis must be weighed very carefully.
• Two large randomized trials have shown that carotid endarterectomy for stenosis $\geq 60 \sim 70\%$ reduces ipsilateral ischemic stroke compared to medical therapy*.
  ■ ACAS showed that the 5-year risk was 5.1% for surgical vs. 11.0% for medical therapy.[59]
  ■ The results were confirmed by the ACST trial, which showed 5-year stroke risk of 6.4% for surgical vs. 11.8% for medical therapy.[60]
  ■ The overall subsequent risk is smaller than that for symptomatic carotid stenosis. The absolute risk reduction is

about 1% per year, with NNT 17–19 to prevent 1 ipsilateral ischemic stroke in 5 years.

- The perioperative risk was 2.3% in ACAS and 3.1% in ACST.
- If one considers surgical treatment for asymptomatic carotid stenosis, the surgeon must have volume and experience.
- Women, for reasons which are unclear, have smaller benefit from carotid endarterectomy than men.

SURGERY: CAROTID STENTING VS. ENDARTERECTOMY

- Carotid stenting, though performed for several years now, is still considered investigational.
- SAPPHIRE was a randomized trial designed to compare carotid stenting (with a distal protection device) to endarterectomy in high-risk patients with symptomatic and asymptomatic carotid stenosis.
  - It showed that the stroke rates at two years are equivalent (stenting is not inferior) and there was a trend favoring stenting in rate of adverse events.[61]
- Several ongoing studies, including CREST, SPACE, EVA-3 S, and CAVATAS-2, are examining the effectiveness of the procedure in stroke prevention. So far, safety appears similar to that of CEA except in patients > 80 years old.
- Some unresolved issues are durability of the stent and re-stenosis rates. The eventual hope is that carotid stenting will be cheaper and safer, especially in those with multiple medical comorbidities.
- Carotid stenting is approved for TIA and stroke patients where the stenosis is hard to reach surgically, where there are medical comorbidities that increase the risk of surgery, or in

cases of post-radiation or postoperative stenoses. Outside of theses situations, stenting should be done only in the context of the aforementioned clinical trials.

WHEN CAN YOU DO SURGERY OR STENTING AFTER A STROKE?

- CEA performed **early** after a symptomatic event confers the greatest benefit since the highest risk of recurrent stroke is in the first two weeks after a TIA or minor stroke.
- Combined data of NASCET and ECST trials show that the benefit of CEA is greatest with CEA performed within two weeks of symptoms.[62,63] These trials, as well as a systematic review, saw no increased risk of early surgery (defined as earlier than 2–6 weeks).[64] However, "unstable symptoms" or "urgent" surgery are also among the strongest risk factors for perioperative complications.
- Traditionally, it has been recommended to wait 4–6 weeks after a large stroke to perform revascularization by CEA. The rationale is that reperfusing an area of recent stroke might lead to hyperperfusion or even hemorrhage. Breakdown of the blood–brain barrier and loss of autoregulation in the area of injury may lead to edema and bleeding. Also, at the time of stroke, it may be unclear how well the patient will recover and how aggressive to be with various prevention strategies.
- In summary, it is probably best to revascularize early (within two weeks), especially after a TIA or if the stroke is small clinically and radiographically. There have been several studies in this regard, but none conclusive. A sense of "urgency" should be tempered with awareness of complications.

■ Acute carotid occlusion

Carotid occlusion can cause a stroke by two mechanisms: hemodynamic reduction of flow or embolism into the downstream cerebral circulation. These two mechanisms can often be distinguished by the appearance of the stroke on MRI, and by perfusion studies. Hemodynamic strokes will have a "watershed" distribution of infarction and reduced flow in the distal beds of the MCA, ACA, and PCA, while emboli will have a classical embolic distribution of infarction and reduced flow in the branches of these vessels.

- Carotid occlusion patients are at high risk for recurrent stroke by either mechanism.
- In general, patients with carotid occlusion are managed conservatively with risk factor reduction, careful maintenance of cerebral perfusion by cautious blood pressure control, and antiplatelet drugs. Aggressive intervention with anticoagulants or revascularization is mainly reserved for patients with small areas of infarction who are having continued symptoms and are at perceived risk of deterioration or recurrence.
- One traditional approach is to anticoagulate acutely and for several months after acute symptomatic carotid occlusion to prevent distal emboli. The thinking has been that the end of the occlusion intracranially has an unstable clot that can propagate or embolize. However, there are no conclusive data supporting anticoagulation and substantial variability exists among stroke experts on this issue, so the decision is usually individualized from patient to patient.
- Carotid occlusion can also be revascularized surgically (by CEA) or endovascularly (by intra-arterial lysis with or without stenting). The clot is usually at the internal carotid origin, and

the rest of the artery downstream might be open. Though acute revascularization has been advocated by some, there are no prospective data to support the theory that acute revascularization (1) improves the patient's symptoms from current stroke or (2) prevents recurrent stroke long-term. There are substantial risks to acute revascularization and such patients must be selected very carefully.

- In the USA there is an ongoing randomized NIH-sponsored trial in patients with chronic carotid occlusion evaluating extracranial–intracranial bypass surgery versus medical therapy (Carotid Occlusion Stroke Study).[65] This surgical therapy tries to augment cerebral perfusion ipsilateral to carotid occlusion by connecting a temporal artery branch of the external carotid artery with the middle cerebral artery.

- If bypass is considered, there are several measurement methods for risk stratification by hemodynamic reserve:
  - Xenon-CT or single photon emission CT (SPECT) with acetazolamide (Diamox) challenge.
  - PET with oxygen extraction fraction.[66]
  - TCD with breath-holding index (BHI).[67]
    - Normal BHI $\geq 0.69 \rightarrow$ <10% ipsilateral stroke in 2 years.
    - Impaired BHI $< 0.69 \rightarrow$ 40% ipsilateral stroke in 2 years.

■ Lacunar strokes

Lacunar strokes, also known as small-vessel disease or small-vessel occlusion, account for approximately 20–30% of strokes. They are due to obstruction of penetrating end arteries off major intracranial arteries (off the MCA, basilar artery, PCA, ACA, and posterior communicating artery). These infarcts are <15 mm diameter in size.

ARE ALL SMALL SUBCORTICAL STROKES < 15 mm LACUNAR STROKES (i.e. DUE TO SMALL-VESSEL DISEASE)?

- No, they are not. 12% of small basal ganglia and 34% of centrum semiovale infarcts have a cardioembolic source, and 19% of small basal ganglia and 53% of centrum semiovale infarcts have large-artery occlusive disease.[68]
- Some are larger than 15 mm and are clearly not in a distribution of a single small arteriole.[69]
- Not all lacunar syndromes (see below) are caused by small strokes.
- Therefore, even a "lacunar-looking" stroke, especially if it does not fit into a classic syndrome or appearance, warrants careful work-up for large-artery atherosclerosis and embolic source.

WHAT CAUSES LACUNAR STROKES?

- Lipohyalinosis is the classic pathology, but atherosclerosis is also a common cause for small-vessel occlusion.
- Seen from an epidemiological standpoint, hypertension is the only consistent risk factor, whereas contributions of diabetes mellitus, smoking, or hyperlipidemia are smaller, if any.
- Antihypertensive treatment is the only method that has been shown to reduce lacunar strokes in particular.[70]

LACUNAR SYNDROMES AND THEIR LOCALIZATION

- Pure motor hemiparesis (corona radiata, anterior or posterior limb of internal capsule, pons, and medullary pyramid).
- Pure sensory stroke (ventral posterior thalamus).

- Sensorimotor stroke (thalamus, corona radiata).
- Ataxic hemiparesis (not well localizing: pons, corona radiata, anterior or posterior limb of internal capsule, lentiform nucleus, cerebellum).
- Dysarthria – clumsy hand (anterior limb of internal capsule, genu, pons).

■ Cervical arterial dissection

Arterial dissection is probably an under-recognized stroke mechanism.

PATHOLOGY

- Dissection occurs due to an intimal tear in the vessel wall and the formation of an intramural hematoma, sometimes associated with a pseudoaneurysm.
- Flow may be obstructed by compression of the lumen by the wall hematoma, or by intraluminal clot.
- Distal embolization from the area of injury downstream into the intracranial circulation is probably the most common stroke mechanism.
- In the internal carotid artery, dissection usually occurs 2 or more cm distal to the carotid bifurcation, and in the vertebral artery at the C1–2 level where the artery leaves the transverse canal of the axis bone. Intracranial dissections can also occur but are less common.
- Neck or head trauma and chiropractic manipulation are known precipitating factors. Motor vehicle accidents with whiplash or seatbelt injuries to the neck are probably the most common cause seen in most hospitals. However, many people with cervical artery dissections do not have clear precipitating events.

- Fibromuscular dysplasia and heritable arteriopathies such as Ehlers–Danlos syndrome predispose to arterial dissections, but most individuals do not have underlying arterial pathology.

DIAGNOSIS

- Ischemic stroke or TIA is the usual presenting symptom.
- A history of neck, facial, or head pain in a patient without strong risk factors for vascular disease points toward the diagnosis.
- Horner's syndrome may occur because of injury to sympathetic fibers lying on the outside of the carotid artery wall.
- Subarachnoid hemorrhage can occur if the dissection occurs or extends intracranially, because there are only two layers in the vessel wall, compared to three extracranially.

TESTING

When dissection is suspected, diagnostic testing should go beyond routine carotid ultrasound and MR angiography. Carotid ultrasound tends to focus at the carotid bifurcation and thus may not detect dissection, which is often located more rostrally. MRA detects large dissections but not a subtle intimal tear and flap.

Better diagnostic tests:

- MRI T1 sequence with fat suppression of the neck – Talk to your radiologist to be sure they know that dissection is suspected. Hematoma in false lumen is bright.
- CT Angiogram – A good CTA can give information similar to DSA.[71]
- Digital subtraction angiogram (DSA) – Find characteristic tapering lumen, rarely pseudoaneurysm, in locations usually not associated with atherosclerosis. Though considered a gold standard, sometimes it is not clear whether the abnormality is due to dissection or atherosclerosis.

Several diagnostic methodologies might be necessary to conclude that an artery has a dissection.

THERAPY

- Anticoagulation for 3–6 months has been the traditional medical therapy, since the mechanism of cerebral infarction is probably most often due to thromboembolism, though there are no randomized trials to support anticoagulation.
- The risk of stroke/TIA recurrence is low (~1.5% per year).[72] Whether antiplatelet agents are sufficient remains uncertain.
- Most of the time, dissected arteries heal over time, leaving variable degrees of residual stenosis.
- Sometimes dissection is treated by endovascular or surgical means, though these interventions are not needed in most cases. The reasons for interventions include expanding pseudoaneurysm, or recurrent symptoms due to either hemodynamically significant stenosis or recurrent embolization. Stents can expand the lumen and detachable coils can be placed in the pseudoaneurysm.

■ Patent foramen ovale

The role of PFO in pathophysiology and prevention of stroke remains controversial.

RELATION TO STROKE

- PFO is detected in 20–30% of the general population.
- PFO is more prevalent (30–50%) among stroke patients who are young and do not have other causes of stroke (cryptogenic, age < 50).

- PFO is most likely causally related to the stroke when the PFO is large and associated with an atrial septal aneurysm.[73]
- PFO is probably not a causal factor for stroke when it is found in a person who has known atherosclerosis, other known stroke mechanism, or is elderly (>60).[74]
- The proposed mechanism relating PFO to ischemic stroke is "paradoxical embolism." Venous thrombus in systemic venous circulation bypasses the pulmonary circulation and embolizes to the brain. Finding deep venous thrombosis in the lower extremities (by ultrasound) or in the pelvic veins (by MRI), or detecting hypercoagulability (factor V Leiden, prothrombin gene mutation, anticardiolipin antibodies etc.) would support this mechanism.
- However, the bottom line is that in the patient you are seeing it is difficult to know whether the PFO is an incidental finding or causally related to stroke.

TREATMENT

- In most patients with stroke and PFO, antiplatelet drugs are sufficient.
- So far the data suggest that anticoagulation does not offer additional benefit over aspirin,[50] unless hypercoagulability or venous thrombosis is found.
- Endovascular closure devices have improved over the past decade and are considered to carry a "low risk." There are randomized trials ongoing which aim to answer the question whether endovascular PFO closure is better than medical therapy in stroke prevention (RESPECT, CLOSURE-I, and PC-Trial).

7

Transient ischemic attack (TIA)

Transient neurological symptoms often present a difficult diagnostic dilemma. It is often difficult to tell if the transient symptoms were due to ischemia or due to something else (see Chapter 1). Usually, by the time the physician sees the patient, the neurological exam has returned to normal.

On the other hand, it is critically important not to miss the diagnosis of TIA. TIAs may provide an opportunity for physicians to intervene and prevent an ischemic stroke and subsequent disability and must be taken seriously. Search for an etiology must be done expeditiously. Just as angina may serve as a warning for future myocardial infarction, a TIA is often a warning sign of an impending stroke.

■ Definition

A transient ischemic attack (TIA) is a brief episode of neurologic dysfunction caused by focal brain or retinal ischemia, with **clinical symptoms typically lasting less than one hour**, and without evidence of acute infarction on brain imaging.[75]

■ Etiology

The causes are the same as for ischemic stroke. Determining the etiology of the ischemic symptoms expeditiously is very important as there are several causes that, if treated urgently, may prevent a stroke. Such causes include atrial fibrillation and symptomatic carotid stenosis.

■ Presentation

TIAs present the same way as an acute ischemic stroke. The only difference is that the symptoms and signs rapidly and completely resolve, usually within minutes. There is not a typical presentation – it depends on the vascular territory affected.

■ Differential diagnosis

- Syncope: look for pre-syncopal symptoms.
- Seizure: ask about prior history of seizure, or if any of the following occurred with the event: shaking, clouding of consciousness, tongue biting, incontinence.
- Migraine: be careful about attributing a TIA or stroke to migraine unless there is a clear history of previous migraine with complicated features similar to this event.
- Vestibular dysfunction; vertigo.
- Anxiety, panic attack.
- Hypoglycemia.
- Drug intoxication.
- Mass such as tumor or subdural hematoma.
- Metabolic encephalopathy.

■ Clinical approach to a patient with suspected TIA

Evaluation of TIA is the same as for ischemic stroke, since the pathophysiology of TIA and ischemic stroke are the same. TIA should be thought of as a briefer, smaller ischemic stroke, but with the same implications for recurrence.

HISTORY AND PHYSICAL EXAM

- Make sure that the neurologic symptoms have resolved!
  - If you document a normal neurological exam and later the patient develops recurrent neurological deficits, they can still be treated with TPA because the clock starts over from the time of new symptoms, as long as the patient was completely back to normal in between.
- Since you are likely to be seeing the patient after, and not during, the TIA, get an objective description as much as possible, perhaps from a witness:
  - "Were you able to move your arm?"
  - "Was his speech slurred?"
  - "Was she able to walk normally?

BRAIN IMAGING

Consider skipping CT and going straight to MRI and MRA if possible.

CT is expected to be normal because

- it was transient ischemia;
  or

- ischemia continues to be present but it's too small to see on CT;

  or
- it was *not* ischemia.

MRI is more likely than CT to be helpful because

- it shows you a small stroke that you didn't see on CT (ischemia improved to make the patient symptomatically back to baseline but tissue was damaged);

  or
- it shows you a vascular lesion that, by association, makes you suspect that it was an ischemic event (small vessel disease, old stroke, arterial stenosis, etc.);

  or
- it shows you some other explanation of the transient event (subdural hematoma, tumor, etc.).

DECIDE WHETHER THIS IS MORE LIKELY A TIA OR SOMETHING ELSE

Other tests might be done to exclude non-TIA diagnoses if they are suspected.

Electrocardiogram (EKG) is helpful because

- if you see atrial fibrillation, it was likely to have been a cardioembolic TIA. In these cases, initiating treatment with anticoagulation may prevent a stroke.

Measurement of blood sugar is helpful because

- hypoglycemia can explain the event.

Measurement of other electrolytes is helpful because

- electrolyte abnormalities may also explain the event.

Table 7.1. The risk of stroke after TIA: the Diabetes, Duration, Weakness (DDW) score.

Three risk factors for stroke after TIA (Give 1 point each if present)	Number of risk factors present	Estimated risk of stroke in 7 days
• Diabetes mellitus	0	1%
• Duration of episode $\geq$ 60 minutes	1	4%
• Weakness (focal) with episode	2	9%
	3	10%

Notes:
(1) These are risk factors that make ischemic etiology more likely.
(2) This prognostication score has not been prospectively validated in an independent dataset.
Adapted from: S. C. Johnston & S. Sidney, Validation of a 4-point prediction rule to stratify short-term stroke risk after TIA. *Stroke* 2005; **36**: 430.[77] Reproduced with permission from Lippincott Williams & Wilkins.

MANAGEMENT

Again, the management is similar to that for acute ischemic stroke, as are the preventive measures.

• Observe the patient for 24 hours. Remember, if they develop new neurological symptoms they could be candidates for TPA if no other exclusions exist.
• Start daily antiplatelets.
• MRI to evaluate for new and old stroke.
• Carotid ultrasound and TCD, MRA of neck and brain, or CT angiogram of neck and brain to look for arterial stenosis. Be sure to evaluate the entire cerebrovascular system.
• EKG, and consider EKG telemetry.
• Cardiovascular risk-factor evaluation of blood pressure, lipids, and fasting glucose.

- Consider echocardiogram for evaluation of cardioembolic source.
- Educate the patient about:
  - stroke risk factors including smoking, exercise, weight loss, alcohol;
  - specific medications prescribed for prevention;
  - recurrent symptoms to look for; and
  - calling emergency services for acute stroke symptoms.
- Discharge with established follow-up plans.

■ Prognosis after TIA

- After an ED visit for TIA:[76]
  - 5.3% stroke risk **within 2 days**;
  - 10.5% stroke in 90 days (21% fatal, 64% disabling).
- 1 in 9 patients will have a stroke within 3 months.
- The key problem is trying to predict who will have a stroke (Table 7.1).

8

Intracerebral hemorrhage (ICH)

In this chapter we will consider spontaneous hemorrhage into the brain parenchyma and ventricles (intracerebral hemorrhage, ICH). Non-traumatic bleeding into the subarachnoid space (subarachnoid hemorrhage, SAH) will be covered in Chapter 9. Traumatic subdural and epidural hemorrhages are not covered in this book.

Intracerebral hemorrhage is associated with very high morbidity and mortality, but it is also very preventable.

■ Definition

Spontaneous bleeding into the brain parenchyma or ventricles from a ruptured artery, vein, or other vascular structure (Fig. 8.1).

It is important to distinguish primary ICH, which is the topic of this chapter, from hemorrhagic transformation of an ischemic infarct, covered in Chapter 5. In primary ICH, the initial event is vascular rupture, while in hemorrhagic transformation the initial event is vascular occlusion. This is obviously an important distinction since the etiologies and treatments are completely different. The term "hemorrhagic stroke" is used loosely and imprecisely and is often applied to either of these conditions. We prefer the more precise distinction.

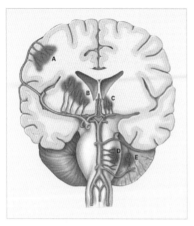

Figure 8.1. Location of hemorrhages. Penetrating cortical branches of the anterior, middle, or posterior cerebral arteries (A); basal ganglia, originating from ascending lenticulostriate branches of the middle cerebral artery (B); the thalamus, originating from ascending thalmogeniculate branches of the posterior cerebral artery (C); the pons, originating from paramedian branches of the basilar artery (D); and the cerebellum, originating from penetrating branches of the posterior inferior, anterior inferior, or superior cerebellar arteries (E).
Source: A. I. Qureshi, S. Tuhrim, J. P. Broderick, H. H. Batjer, H. Hondo, & D. F. Hanley, Spontaneous intracerebral hemorrhage. *N. Engl. J. Med.* 2001; **344**: 1450–60.[78]
Reproduced with permission. Copyright © 2001 Massachusetts Medical Society.

■ Etiology

- Hypertension (most common).
  - Classic locations for hypertensive intracerebral hemorrhage:
    - basal ganglia (putamen most common)
    - thalamus

- pons
- cerebellum
- Amyloid angiopathy – More often cortical in location than hypertensive hemorrhages.
- Drugs:
  - iatrogenic, i.e., heparin or coumadin
  - drugs of abuse, especially cocaine
- Vascular malformation (aneurysm, AVM, cavernous angioma).
- Cerebral vein thrombosis – Caused by bleeding from congested vein feeding into an occluded cortical vein or venous sinus thrombosis, this may technically be considered transformation of a "venous infarct". However, an underlying infarct is not necessarily present or may be very minor, and the clinical presentation of the thrombosis may be dominated by the development of ICH. This is different from arterial occlusion and hemorrhagic transformation, where the initial clinical presentation is almost always the result of the infarct, and the hemorrhage comes hours later.
- Tumor.
- Trauma.

■ Presentation

You cannot distinguish ICH from ischemic stroke on the basis of the clinical presentation – they may look exactly alike. This is the reason brain imaging is so critical in initial stroke management, since brain bleeding can readily be detected by CT or MRI immediately after it occurs.

Clinical features that might suggest ICH rather than an infarct include accelerated hypertension, vomiting (always a bad sign in an acute stroke patient, usually indicative of increasing ICP), or decreasing level of consciousness.

■ Diagnosis and evaluation

As with ischemic stroke, management in the first few hours may make the difference between a good and bad outcome.

INITIAL ASSESSMENT

- History and physical exam.
  - Look for signs of trauma.
- Glasgow coma scale (GCS) and brainstem reflexes if comatose, NIHSS score if awake.
- Measure blood pressure (see subsequent comment for details on blood-pressure management).
- Oxygen saturation.
  - Consider intubation for airway protection.
- CT.
  - Repeat CT if patient was transferred from outside hospital (the bleed could have extended en route).
  - Where did the bleed start?
  - Is there significant mass effect, intraventricular hemorrhage (IVH), or hydrocephalus?
- Measure the volume (diameter A × diameter B × C)/2.
  - C = number of slices that show hemorrhage × thickness of the slice.
  - (see also Appendix 1, Numbers and calculations).
- Check platelet count, INR, and PTT, and urine drug screen.
- EKG: rule out MI.
  - Consider cardiac enzymes.

- Consider vascular study (MRA, CTA, or DSA) to rule out AVM or aneurysm.
  - Especially if:
    - younger patient; or
    - there is SAH present; or
    - ICH in an atypical lobar or cortical location, or with some other atypical appearance.
- Consider MRI:
  - To look for multiple old hemorrhages or microbleeds that might suggest amyloid angiopathy.
  - To exclude underlying tumor.
  - To check for venous thrombosis (order MR venogram if suspected):
    - hemorrhages high in convexity, often bilateral, with substantial edema.
- Consider getting neurosurgery consult (see **Surgical intervention**, below):
  - for possible hematoma evacuation or ventriculostomy;
  - if aneurysm or AVM suspected.

■ Management

It is important to talk with family and start the process of coming to terms with the often poor prognosis (see **Prognosis and outcome**, below). This is a very important management consideration. Discuss "Do Not Resuscitate" (DNR) issues. However, in the first day, don't be too certain of bad outcome unless herniation has already occurred. Comatose patients can wake up, especially if the mass effect is decompressed spontaneously into the ventricle, or by surgical intervention. Do not withdraw support in the ED.

SURGICAL INTERVENTION

- Surgical evacuation of hematoma is to prevent death from mass effect.
  - There is no evidence that routine surgical clot evacuation results in improved outcome (ISTICH trial).[79*]
- Surgical clot evacuation is usually reserved for patients with the following:[79,80*]
  - Younger age: no absolute cutoff but almost certainly < 75 years.
  - Cerebellar hemorrhages with:
    - displacement of fourth ventricle;
    - enlargement of temporal horns (early obstructive hydrocephalus);
    - compression of brainstem;
    - decreased level of consciousness (but don't wait until the patient is comatose if above criteria are met).
  - Supratentorial hemorrhages with:
    - superficial location: close to brain surface;
    - volume > 20 cc;
    - drowsy but not comatose;
    - more likely if not in eloquent location.
- Ventriculostomy and CSF drainage:
  - May be life-saving if obstructive hydrocephalus is present.

HEMATOMA ENLARGEMENT

- Occurs in 20–35% of ICH:[81]
  - all locations;
  - usually in the first few hours after onset of symptoms but almost always in the first 24 hours;

- may occur later in patients with coagulopathy (coumadin);
  - associated with much worse prognosis.
- Aggressive blood-pressure reduction to SBP ≤ 150, MAP 100–110 may reduce hemorrhage enlargement (see below).
  - unproven (trials ongoing).
- Activated factor VII (NovoSeven).
  - Recent phase II trial data suggest that hemorrhage growth can be prevented by giving activated factor VII, 40–160 µg/kg.[82]
  - This drug (NovoSeven) is expensive and can have dose-related occlusive complications such as stroke, myocardial infarction, pulmonary embolism, etc.
  - Pending further data and recommendations, we are using this drug (80 µg/kg, single dose IV) in patients with ICH if it can be started within four hours of symptom onset or if the ICH is associated with coagulopathy (see next section). Patients with associated arterial occlusive diseases (coronary or cerebral ischemia, peripheral vascular disease, or pulmonary embolus), or who have already herniated, are not considered.

WARFARIN (COUMADIN)-RELATED INTRACEREBRAL HEMORRHAGE

Goal: normal INR using fresh frozen plasma (FFP) 20 mL/kg and vitamin K*

- CT brain immediately.
- INR, PTT, thrombin time, D-dimers, fibrinogen, CBC.
- Type and cross, order 4 units of fresh frozen plasma (FFP).
- Give vitamin K 10 mg IV over 10 minutes AND half of FFP (10 mL/kg). One unit of FFP = 200–250 mL. Give diuretics if needed.

- Repeat INR and FFP 10 mL/kg every 20–30 minutes until INR is normalized.
- Activated factor VII (NovoSeven) (see above). Dose may be reduced to 20–40 µg/kg and repeated.

HEPARIN-RELATED INTRACEREBRAL HEMORRHAGE

- Stop heparin.
- CT brain immediately.
- INR, PTT, platelets, CBC, fibrinogen, thrombin time, D-dimers.
- Type and cross.
- Give protamine: 25 mg initial dose; check stat PTT 10 minutes later and if increased give 10 mg additionally; repeat until PTT normal.*

WHAT IS THE TARGET BLOOD PRESSURE AFTER ICH?

Does lowering blood pressure cause ischemia or reduce the risk of rebleeding?

- The simple answer is that we don't know. There is a debate as to whether there is an ischemic region around the hematoma. Various studies using various techniques have resulted in conflicting data, but the general consensus is that ischemia is not a major cause of damage except with very large hematomas. The consensus is that it is safe to lower a very high blood pressure.
- The risk of hematoma enlargement has been associated with increasing BP, with decreased risk associated with systolic blood pressures (SBP) ≤ 150 mm Hg, but whether lowering the blood pressure reduces the risk is unknown.

- The AHA/ASA guidelines recommend mean blood pressure (MAP) goal of 130 mm Hg* but it is poor-quality evidence (level of evidence V, grade C recommendation).[80] It is possible that lower MAP (e.g., around 110 mm Hg) would result in better outcome, but this remains to be tested.
- **Until we have more data, we tend to be aggressive in lowering SBP to 150 and MAP to 100–120 mm Hg in the first 12–24 hours post-ICH.**
  - Use titratable drugs such as nicardipine and labetalol:
    - nicardipine 5 mg/hr and titrate up to 15 mg/hr as needed;
    - labetalol 10–20 mg IV bolus, repeat as needed up to 60 mg.
  - Avoid nitroprusside.
  - Other antihypertensive agents are usually not effective in the ED for accelerated hypertension associated with ICH.

ICH SUBSEQUENT CARE

- Continue to control blood pressure but maintain CPP > 70 mm Hg.
- Goal ICP < 20 mm Hg:
  - Ventricular drainage.
  - Ventricular drainage recently coupled with instillation of thrombolytics into the ventricle to accelerate ventricular clot dissolution and drainage of CSF (unproven – trials under way).
- Maintain euvolemia, normothermia.
- Watch for neurologic deterioration (see below).
- Withhold all antithrombotic drugs for 2 weeks.
  - Compression stockings to prevent DVT.
  - Uncertain when to start DVT prophylaxis with SC heparin or low molecular weight heparin, but probably wait at least 24 hours to be sure that no hemorrhagic enlargement is occurring and that coagulation parameters are normalized.

- Talk with family about expected quality of life, advanced directives, withdrawal of support if appropriate.
- Start working on **disposition** early: rehab consult, case manager.

■ Prognosis and outcome

NEUROLOGIC DETERIORATION IN ICH

(the ranking is **our impression**):

Cause 1: rebleeding.

Cause 2: hydrocephalus (might itself be due to rebleeding).

Cause 3: cerebral edema.

Cause 4: general medical problems (infection, MI, electrolyte imbalance, pulmonary emboli).

ICH OUTCOME

Correlates with initial GCS, size of hematoma, and presence of IVH.[83]

- GCS < 9 and ICH volume > 60 cc: 90% 1-month mortality
- GCS ≥ 9 and ICH volume < 30 cc: 17% 1-month mortality

Also see the **ICH score** in Appendix 14.[84]

- ICH score ≥ 5: close to 100% 1-month mortality
- ICH score ≥ 4: > 90% 1-month mortality
- ICH score = 2: 20–30% 1-month mortality
- ICH score ≤ 1: < 15% 1-month mortality

But also remember that it can be a "self-fulfilling prophecy." If one treats with the expectation that the patient will do badly, the patient will do badly.

9

Subarachnoid hemorrhage (SAH)

This chapter will discuss the diagnosis and management of spontaneous subarachnoid hemorrhage due to rupture of intracranial aneurysms. The end of the chapter will also discuss unruptured intracranial aneurysms. Much SAH management is not based on good-quality evidence. Much of what is recommended here comes from published practice guidelines and what is commonly practiced.[85] Options for therapy might be limited by the availability and experience of persons performing surgery, endovascular therapy, and neurointensive care.

■ Definition

Subarachnoid hemorrhage is bleeding into the subarachnoid space around the brain. **Trauma** is the most common cause of SAH. We will not discuss traumatic SAH in this chapter. This chapter will discuss **spontaneous SAH**, 80% of which are due to intracranial saccular aneurysms.

■ Epidemiology

- 3% of all strokes but 5% of stroke deaths.
- Incidence 6–15 per 100 000 person years in the USA, with higher risk among African-Americans. Worldwide, higher incidence reported in Japan and Scandinavia.

- Females have higher incidence (60% of patients are female).
- Risk factors: tobacco use, oral contraceptives, alcohol, and stimulants.
- Other disease associated with aneurysms: polycystic kidney disease, Marfan's syndrome, Ehlers–Danlos syndrome, coarctation of the aorta, fibromuscular dysplasia.
- Location: 30% anterior communicating, 25% posterior communicating, 20% MCAs, 10% basilar, 5% vertebral, and 25% have multiple aneurysms.

■ Presentation

- "The worst headache of my life".
- "Thunder-clap headache".
- Headache is sometimes associated with focal neurologic symptoms.

■ Diagnosis

As this condition is potentially life-threatening, diagnostic evaluation should be done emergently.

DIAGNOSIS OF SUBARACHNOID HEMORRHAGE

- CT of the head without contrast.
  - If head CT is normal, but you have a high clinical suspicion for SAH, you **must** do a lumbar puncture, because CT can miss small or subtle SAHs, especially if more than 72 hours has passed since the ictus.
- Lumbar puncture.
  - Don't forget to personally examine the fluid for xanthochromia. Compare the color to water. Measure red blood

cells in first and last tube collected. Also, it is often helpful to personally deliver the tubes of CSF to the lab to make sure that they are processed quickly.

DIAGNOSIS OF INTRACRANIAL ANEURYSMS

- Digital subtraction angiography (DSA): the gold standard.
- CT angiography: quite good, but depends on CT equipment. Difficult to see aneurysms near bones.
- MRA: fair test for screening for unruptured aneurysms > 5 mm.

CAUSES OF SAH OTHER THAN INTRACRANIAL ANEURYSM

- Perimesencephalic SAH: blood limited to anterior to midbrain (or pons). Angiogram is normal. The cause of bleed is unknown (venous?). It carries a good prognosis and benign course.
- Arteriovenous malformation (AVM): it classically causes intra-parenchymal hemorrhage, but it can lead to SAH. DSA will help in diagnosis.
- Arterial dissection (vertebral artery usually): arterial dissection that extends from the extracranial to the intracranial portion of an artery or is limited to the intracranial artery can lead to SAH. This can occur spontaneously or post-traumatic. DSA and MRI can be helpful in visualizing the abnormality.
- Arteriovenous fistula: can be seen only with careful DSA.
- Pituitary apoplexy: MRI is helpful in making the diagnosis.
- Cocaine: can lead to SAH, ICH, or cerebral ischemia.
- Trauma: detailed history or external head examination may suggest trauma as the primary cause.
- Vasculitis: difficult to diagnose, since DSA is neither sensitive nor specific and brain biopsy is specific but insensitive.

■ Ruptured aneurysms: management

GOALS

- Prevention of rebleeding.
- Treatment of the aneurysm itself: clip or coil.
- Prevention and treatment of complications: hydrocephalus, seizure, vasospasm, hyponatremia, infections, and DVTs.
- Rehabilitation (see Chapter 11).

PREVENTION OF REBLEEDING

Rebleeding is maximal in the first 24 hours after SAH (4%). It carries a high mortality.

The following measures are often performed, but without much evidence:

- Blood pressure control may be important before definitive treatment to reduce rebleeding.
- Bed rest in ICU with monitoring.
- Anti-fibrinolytic drugs (epsilon amino caproic acid, tanxemic acid) reduce rebleeding but promote ischemic complications.* Consequently these drugs are rarely used.

TREATMENT OF THE ANEURYSM ITSELF

It should be done as early as possible, especially in patients with mild to moderate clinical deficits, since the goal is to prevent rebleeding.

Surgical clipping*
Craniotomy and placement of metal clip takes the aneurysm out of the arterial circulation.

- It is believed to be the best way to prevent aneurysmal bleeding long-term.
- **But** it carries morbidity, and some aneurysms are not amenable to clipping due to location, shape, etc.

Endovascular coiling*

Coiling has become the alternative treatment. When you fill the aneurysm with coils, it thromboses, and effectively takes the aneurysm out of the arterial circulation.

- Subsequent rebleed rate is not as low as with surgical clipping, but pretty close.
- This procedure may not be as durable as clipping. Long-term data are not available. Also, complete obliteration of the aneurysm is not always achieved initially and may require repeat intervention.
- Some aneurysms are not amenable to coiling due to distal location or shape.

Clipping or coiling?

That is the big question.

- It appears that endovascular coiling carries lower morbidity than surgical clipping.
- ISAT was a randomized multi-center trial comparing the two methods:[86]
  - 23.7% of coiled vs. 30.6% of clipped patients were dependent or dead at 1 year (absolute risk reduction of a bad outcome: 6.9%).
  - For this trial, the patients were required to be good candidates for both procedures (~60% were treated outside the trial). 88% of patients had mild SAH (World Federation of Neurological Surgeons grade 1 or 2; see Appendix 14).

- Locations: 51% were anterior cerebral or anterior communicating artery (ACA/AcomA) and 33% were ICA or posterior communicating artery (PcomA) aneurysms. Only 14% were MCA aneurysms and 2.7% were posterior circulation aneurysms.
- Based on ISAT, the preferred treatment of ruptured ACA, ICA, anterior or posterior communicating artery aneurysms is coiling. The preferred modality for treatment of ruptured posterior circulation aneurysm (i.e., basilar artery aneurysm) in many centers is coiling. For distal MCA aneurysms, some may be difficult to approach by coiling and need to be clipped.

PREVENTION AND TREATMENT OF COMPLICATIONS

As with other strokes, general medical complications such as DVT, pneumonia, and other infection are common. SAH has particular complications that we will address here: hydrocephalus, seizure, cerebral vasospasm and delayed ischemic deficits.

Hydrocephalus

Hydrocephalus occurs in ~20% of patients with SAH. This may be already present at the time of presentation with SAH.

Diagnosis

- Clinical signs include a decrease in level of consciousness, agitation, hypertension, and bradycardia. However, these signs are not specific.
- CT of head without contrast: enlargement of ventricles.

Treatment

- External drainage of CSF via intraventricular catheter (ventriculostomy or external ventricular drain).
- Ventriculostomy must be monitored for amount of CSF drained and for infection.
- If hydrocephalus is persistent, CSF drainage can be converted to internal drainage by placement of ventriculo-peritoneal, ventriculo-atrial, or lumbo-peritoneal shunt by a neurosurgeon.

Seizure

Seizure may increase blood pressure and may increase rebleeding risk.

Prevention

- Without good evidence for efficacy, the current practice is to routinely administer antiepileptic agents to prevent seizures.
- Phenytoin 300 mg per day and adjusted to maintain level of 10–20 μg/mL.

Diagnosis

- Non-convulsive seizure may go unrecognized. Bedside EEG may help if SAH itself or sedative drugs affect assessment.

Treatment

- Phenytoin is most commonly used and is available in intravenous and oral formulations. Among other anticonvulsants, valproic acid and phenobarbital are available in IV formulation.

Cerebral vasospasm and delayed ischemic deficits
- Onset usually 3–5 days after SAH, maximal at 5–10 days.
- ~30% of SAH patients develop vasospasm, and 15–20% go on to have ischemic strokes.

Prevention
- Calcium channel blockers: nimodipine (Nimotop) 60 mg PO every 4 hours × 3 weeks*, but adjust dose downwards if blood pressure falls so low that adequate CPP is endangered. This should be started early after diagnosis of SAH to prevent vasospasm.
- Magnesium: phase II data suggest that magnesium sulfate started within 4 days after SAH and given continuously until 14 days after aneurysm treatment may reduce delayed ischemic deficits.[87] The dose used was magnesium sulfate 64 mmol/L per day with aim of magnesium level of 1.0–2.0 mmol/L.

Diagnosis
- TCD: Velocity trend with daily or sequential measurements is more useful than one-time snapshot of velocities. So get a baseline and follow daily. Lindegaard ratio is the velocity ratio of MCA to extracranial ICA. Increasing flow velocity may indicate either vasospasm or overall increased blood flow. Increasing Lindegaard ratio may be more reliable sign of MCA vasospasm.
- CTA: CT angiography requires iodine contrast injection but may be combined with CT perfusion to diagnose vasospasm and ischemia.
- Angiography: more invasive, but can also be linked to treatment with angioplasty or intra-arterial papaverine.

- Clinical symptoms and signs: similar to ischemic stroke, though in addition may have bilateral frontal lobe dysfunction in the case of anterior communicating artery vasospasm. You want to diagnose and treat vasospasm before these symptoms and signs develop.

Treatment
- Hypertension–hypervolemia–hemodilution (HHH): commonly used. Combination of pressors and volume expanders such as albumin, synthetic starches, colloid, blood.
- Direct endovascular treatment can be performed with balloon angioplasty or drug infusion of papaverine or nicardipine.

■ Prognosis

Mortality: in a population-based study, 3% died before reaching medical attention and one-third died in the first month.[88] A quarter of the deaths are attributable to initial bleed directly, another quarter to vasospasm, and another quarter to rebleeding.
- Morbidity: one-third had neurologic deficit.
- Rebleeding risk: with unclipped aneurysm, 6% rebleed within first 3 days, and 12% in the first 2 weeks.[89] Hypertension increases chance of rebleeding.

■ Admission sequence

Since these patients are usually admitted to Neurosurgery, we are not providing sample admission orders, but do provide the usual sequence of events upon admitting a patient with SAH.

Table 9.1. One-month outcome after SAH by clinical status at presentation, a population-based study.[88]

Clinical status at presentation		Poor outcome (severe neurologic deficits, vegetative, or dead)	Relative risk of poor outcome (95% CI)
Hunt & Hess scale	Grade I	22%	1
	Grade II	22%	1.0 (0.4–2.2)
	Grade III	50%	2.2 (1.1–10.9)
	Grade IV	87%	3.9 (2.3–7.8)
	Grade V	100%	∞
Glasgow coma scale	13–15	24%	1
	9–12	84%	3.6 (2.4–5.2)
	3–8	97%	4.1 (2.9–5.8)

Source: W. T. Longstreth Jr., L. M. Nelson, T. D. Koepsell, & G. van Belle, Clinical course of spontaneous subarachnoid hemorrhage: a population-based study in King County, Washington. *Neurology* 1993; **43**: 712–18.[88] Reproduced with permission from Lippincott Williams & Wilkins.

- Establish diagnosis of SAH with CT or lumbar puncture as soon as possible.
- Neurosurgery consult, admission to ICU.
  - If necessary, transfer emergently to an appropriate hospital that has adequate neurosurgical, neurointerventional (coiling), and neurocritical care capability.
  - Consider ventriculostomy if hydrocephalus is present.
- Determine location of ruptured aneurysm with CT angiogram or digital subtraction angiography (do in the first day).
- Definitive aneurysm treatment (coiling or clipping).

- Nimodipine per nasogastric tube.
- Watch for vasospasm (first 2 weeks).

■ Unruptured aneurysms

Unruptured aneurysms are sometimes found incidentally as part of brain imaging or due to neurologic symptoms other than rupture and SAH. Some patients with SAH are found to have other aneurysms that have not ruptured. Some unruptured aneurysms are found due to screening of those with family history of SAH.

DIAGNOSIS

The diagnostic strategy is the same as for ruptured aneurysms, with DSA being the gold standard for accurate diagnosis and measurement of an aneurysm. CT angiography and MRA are fair screening tools.

NATURAL HISTORY

0.5–1% of the general population harbor unruptured intracranial aneurysms.

Controversy exists among experts about the natural course and decision to intervene.[90,91]

ISUIA study

- The rupture rates were higher for aneurysms of larger size, in the posterior circulation (posterior communicating, posterior cerebral, vertebral, or basilar artery), and in patients with a history of previous SAH.

- Among those with no history of SAH:
  - bleed rate ~0.1% per year if <7 mm diameter.
  - bleed rate ~0.5% per year if 7–12 mm diameter in anterior circulation.
  - bleed rate ~3% per year if 7–12 mm diameter in posterior circulation.
  - bleed rate >3% per year if >12 mm diameter.

Other observational studies
- 1–2% per year.

The controversy and uncertainty of management depends on the paradoxical observation that despite the low rates of rupture of small aneurysms when followed over time, most subarachnoid hemorrhages are due to small aneurysms.

MANAGEMENT

Decision to clip or coil an **unruptured** aneurysm depends on five main factors:
- Previous history of bleeding – increases risk of recurrence and weighs in favor of intervention, either clipping or coiling.
- Aneurysm location – anterior circulation has less rupture risk and has less surgical morbidity.
- Aneurysm size – unruptured aneurysms larger than 7 mm are more likely to bleed.
- Patient age – increased morbidity with any intervention with increased age. Morbidity risk associated with coiling appears to be less dependent on age.
- Surgical experience – perioperative and peri-coiling morbidity is lower in experienced hands.

Treatment decisions for each patient must be individualized by neurology, neurosurgery, and endovascular consultants based on these five variables. We are awaiting definitive data from ongoing trials that will provide more information to assist in our decisions, but the following are "general" recommendations:

- Unruptured aneurysm cavernous or < 5–7 mm: **leave alone**.
- Unruptured aneurysm > 7 mm, anterior circulation, patient < 65 years old, experienced surgeon/center: **surgical clipping**.
- Unruptured aneurysm > 7 mm, posterior circulation, patient > 65 years old, experienced endovascular team: **coiling**.

10

Organization of stroke care

As stroke therapies develop, the context in which stroke care is provided is becoming more important. Creating and maintaining a good organization of stroke care within a region or even a hospital requires much commitment and effort. The European Stroke Initiative provides a good set of evidence-based recommendations.[92,93] An American Stroke Association task force recently published a set of recommendations on systems of stroke care.[94]

■ Timely care

Time is emerging as an important factor in improving outcome. IV TPA must be given within 3 hours, with better results the earlier it is administered. Most investigational stroke therapies for both ischemic and hemorrhagic strokes are focusing on early therapies. A number of important points arise:

- Promotion of public awareness. Patients, family and the general public must be educated regarding stroke symptom recognition, available stroke therapies, and the importance of emergency medical care.
- Education of prehospital providers. Dispatch personnel, ambulance drivers, emergency medical technicians,

paramedics, and their medical supervisors must agree
to prioritize acute stroke and train to increase stroke
recognition.
- Coordination of speedy triage and evaluation. Acute
  stroke patients must be evaluated in a timely fashion, and
  preferentially transported to a stroke center if one is available. In Houston, prehospital providers notify the receiving
  facility or stroke team directly and shorten the time to evaluation. Emergency department physicians should evaluate
  immediately after patient arrival. Stroke team members
  should be notified at the earliest yet most practical time
  possible.
- Stroke team. The establishment of a specialized stroke team
  helps in concentrating expertise and improving the availability of acute stroke care.

■ Stroke units

Specialized stroke units have been shown to improve outcome.[95]* Therefore, all acute stroke patients should ideally be
admitted to a stroke unit. Some uncertainty exists regarding
what features of the stroke unit are important.
- Comprehensive stroke units should have trained
  nurses, therapists (physical, occupational, speech), and
  physicians acting in a multidisciplinary approach.
  This type of stroke unit has been shown to improve
  outcome.*
- Acute stroke care units in the North American model can take
  care of TPA-treated patients. This includes frequent monitoring of vital signs, cardiac rhythm monitoring, and the
  ability to administer some intravenous antihypertensive
  drugs.

■ Stroke centers

Whenever possible, stroke patients should be treated in hospitals with the ability to deliver stroke therapy. It is important to foster the development of such "stroke centers". This may involve the need to establish a regional organization of stroke care.

- Primary stroke centers. There is a need for the establishment of facilities that can provide good basic acute stroke care, with acute stroke teams, stroke units, and ability to administer IV TPA. In the USA the Brain Attack Coalition has published criteria for primary stroke centers,[96] and the Joint Commission on Accreditation of Healthcare Organizations has started accreditation of primary stroke centers (www.jointcommission.org).
- Comprehensive stroke centers would have advanced capability with availability of interventionalists and neurosurgeons.
- Quality assurance measures such as written protocols, and performance measurements should be part of stroke centers.

■ Stroke teams

Acute stroke teams help provide the above care based on the latest evidence-based guidelines. The team might consist of neurologists, internists, emergency department physicians, neurosurgeons, intensivists, rehabilitation physicians, endovascular neurointerventionalists, ultrasonographers, nurses, therapists, dieticians, patient care managers, smoking cessation counselors, stroke educators, etc. Stroke care should be optimized to meet the needs of the local region and institution.

- Acute stroke care might be provided by a mobile stroke team going to different hospitals in a city or region.
- Care might be enhanced by providing streamlined access to a central stroke center.
- In rural areas where physicians with expertise in stroke are often many miles away, consultation by telephone or with advanced telecommunication methods might allow safe administration of thrombolytics locally and facilitate transfer to a stroke center.

11

Rehabilitation

Stroke rehabilitation begins during the acute hospitalization once the patient is medically and neurologically stable. Rehabilitation of the stroke patient with involvement of a multidisciplinary rehabilitation team early during the care of the stroke patient is one of the critical components of stroke unit care that results in improved outcome and shortened length of stay. While practices vary between countries and among hospitals, at our hospital and most stroke centers in the USA the major focus of rehabilitative efforts occurs after the stay in the acute stroke unit, and is beyond the scope of this book. We will focus on those aspects of rehabilitation care that are relevant to acute stroke management in the USA.

The primary goals of rehabilitation are to prevent complications, minimize impairments, and maximize function. The priorities of early stroke rehabilitation are secondary stroke prevention, management of comorbidities and prevention of complications.

The principles of rehabilitation are the same in patients with cerebral infarction and in those with hemorrhage.

TAKE-HOME MESSAGES

- Adequate secondary stroke prevention regimen.
- Prevention of medical complications.

- Early assessment of rehabilitation needs, utilizing a multi-disciplinary rehabilitation team.
- Early initiation of rehabilitation therapies, and greater intensity of therapy, as tolerated by the patient.

■ Secondary stroke prevention

Please see Chapter 6 for detailed discussion.

■ Prevention of medical complications

Please see Appendix 9 for detailed discussion.

■ Multidisciplinary rehabilitation team

The main components of the rehabilitation team are speech therapy, physical therapy, occupational therapy, and psycho-social therapy.

SPEECH THERAPY (ST)

Speech therapy in the stroke unit has two main components: assessment of swallowing and assessment of language function.

Swallowing

The need for swallowing assessment has already been addressed in describing the routine care of the patient with infarct and hemorrhage (Chapter 3). Dysphagia (difficulty with swallowing) is common, occurring in 30–65% of post-stroke patients.[97] Dysphagia may cause malnutrition, dehydration, and aspiration pneumonia.

A bedside swallowing screen should be carried out in all patients before allowing them to eat. If patients are unable to swallow effectively within 12–24 hours, a nasogastric tube (NGT) should be placed for enteral feeding. In fully conscious patients with hemispheric stroke, generally, this can be removed and the patient fed by mouth within several days. If there is any question, a modified barium swallow (MBS) should be completed to assess for aspiration and the patient's ability to safely swallow food and liquids of varying consistencies.

However, many stroke patients have prolonged dysphagia. Most often this occurs in patients with brainstem strokes or with hemispheric stroke associated with depressed level of consciousness, dementia, or confusion. In these cases, a percutaneous endoscopic gastrostomy (PEG) tube should be placed.

Generally, we wait 5 days or so after the stroke before deciding to place a PEG, though in patients who will obviously need one, there is no reason to wait. Begin the process of planning for a PEG early since it takes several days to arrange. Antiplatelet or anticoagulation therapy will raise concerns of bleeding risk and should be addressed as early as possible so as not to delay PEG placement. In our hospital, the procedure can be done by gastroenterologists, general surgeons, or interventional radiologists.

Language

A description of the different aphasic syndromes is beyond the scope of this book. Most stroke patients have non-fluent-type aphasias, where their speech output is reduced or absent, with comprehension being variably affected. It is less common to see pure fluent aphasias affecting only comprehension, though this certainly can occur. Aphasia, especially impaired comprehension, can seriously impede other aspects of rehabilitation since the patient often cannot understand commands of therapists.

As with other aspects of stroke recovery, practice and time with ST will result in at least some improvement in language function, with comprehension usually improving first. Pharmacotherapy with amphetamines, cholinergic, and dopaminergic agents may provide benefit for particular aphasic syndromes but is unproven. The patient's and the family's frustration with impaired ability to communicate should be dealt with in a supportive manner until improvement begins to occur.

PHYSICAL THERAPY (PT)

Physical therapy focuses on bed mobility, transfers, balance, gait training, training to regain normal movement patterns, and wheelchair mobility. Generally, gait training is not begun in earnest until the patient moves off the stroke unit and onto the rehabilitation unit.

In the first few hours after stroke, especially if the patient is fluctuating, we recommend bed rest, keeping the head no higher than 15–30° in order to optimize cerebral perfusion. At the same time, early mobilization is important to prevent deconditioning and deep venous thrombosis. Therefore, we often qualify the bed rest order to allow the patient up with physical therapy and nursing attendance. When the patient first gets up in these cases, the physical therapist and nurse should be instructed to measure the blood pressure before and after sitting and standing, and to maintain careful neurological monitoring, to be sure that the blood pressure doesn't fall or the patient deteriorate.

In the stroke unit, the day following admission, the physical therapist will begin to deal with sitting and transferring from bed to chair, and then standing by the bedside. It is important to remember that patients may have impaired balance and generalized weakness, even if they don't demonstrate a hemiparesis or other signs of weakness or ataxia when lying in bed. Therefore, **every stroke patient should be considered a fall risk when they first get out of bed and should not be allowed up unassisted until evaluated by PT**. This occurs for several reasons. Even a day or two lying in bed can result in a general deconditioning that can lead to generalized weakness and orthostatic hypotension. This can be aggravated by antihypertensive and other medications that are well tolerated when the patient is lying flat, but can cause orthostatic changes when the patient gets out of bed.

80% of stroke patients will eventually regain their ability to walk independently, so that tempered optimism is a reasonable approach when dealing with patients and families in the first few days, even in the case of those with hemiplegia.

OCCUPATIONAL THERAPY (OT)

Occupational therapy focuses on fine and gross motor coordination (pinch, opposition, finger to nose, rapid alternating movements), strength (active range of motion, passive range of motion), tone, sensation, activities of daily living (grooming, bathing, upper extremity dressing, lower extremity dressing, commode transfer, toileting) and training to regain normal movement patterns.

Various assistive devices such as braces and splints may be used to help with supporting weak limbs, stabilizing joints, and avoiding contractures and pressure sores caused by spasticity and immobility. Larger more easily grasped appliances can be used to augment the functional use of a weak limb. The use of these devices is beyond the scope of this chapter.

An important principle of OT is compensation vs. facilitation. Put simplistically, compensation refers to training the unaffected limb to compensate by carrying out functions of the impaired limb, while facilitation refers to repetitive use of the affected limb in order to accelerate recovery and avoid "learned non-use" that might result from over-compensatory reliance on the unaffected limb. Recent animal and human brain mapping studies have shown unexpected cortical plasticity in areas adjacent to the stroke, and even contralateral brain areas, in response to repeated attempts to move an affected limb or digit or, in the case of an aphasic patient, to talk. The observation of increased metabolic activity in these areas not normally associated with the function of the affected limb or language has stimulated renewed interest in early and intensive rehabilitation efforts.

PSYCHOSOCIAL EVALUATION

It is never too early to begin to educate the patient and family about lifestyle changes and medical treatments to prevent another stroke. These need to be reinforced throughout the hospital and rehabilitation stay.

After a major stroke, both the family and the patient go through a grief reaction which at first includes denial and disbelief, and sometimes anger. In particular, the need to insert a PEG is often a crisis point when the family finally comes to terms with the severe disability and prolonged recovery that lies ahead. At this stage, which is usually when the patient is in the acute stroke unit, mainly supportive measures are indicated. More detailed teaching and coping with the consequences of the disability usually waits until after the acute stroke stay when the realities of the impairment become more clear, and the shock, disorientation, and confusion have worn off. Even in patients fully recovering from their stroke, the threat of another event and the realization of vulnerability usually cause significant emotional consequences.

Depression in the patient and caregiver are common. Incontinence is an important contributor to depression and dependence, in addition to the obvious other causes (paralysis, inability to talk, and pain). Pre-morbid depressive tendencies are often amplified after a stroke, so that even patients with little disability may become depressed. Stroke location may also play a role, with more depression reported in non-dominant frontal lesions. Depressed patients often respond well to pharmacotherapy, but again, these psychosocial issues are usually addressed after the acute stroke stay.

The most pressing psychosocial issues to consider in the first few days after stroke onset concern the management of either confusion/delirium or decreased level of arousal.

Delirium

Management of the confused and delirious patient with choice of sedating drugs has been addressed in Chapter 5. Basic rules:
- Sedate only when necessary.
  - Avoid benzodiazepines.
  - Haloperidol (Haldol) 0.5–4 mg PO or IV every 6 hours, risperidone (Risperdal) 0.5–1 mg PO at bedtime or twice daily, quetiapine (Seroquel) 25–50 mg PO once or twice daily, and ziprasidone (Geodon) 10–20 mg IM/PO once or twice daily are probably best.
- Use soft restraints and move to a private room if possible.

Level of arousal

Decreased level of arousal is commonly seen in large hemispheric strokes, and often impedes participation in rehabilitation. Such patients may benefit from activating or stimulant drugs. Pharmacotherapy is usually not initiated before a week post-stroke. It is important to be sure that the patient is not sleepy due to metabolic abnormalities or increased ICP (see Chapter 5).

Amantadine (Symmetrel)

- Dosage: 100 mg morning and noon (initial).
- Contraindications: epilepsy, any seizure disorder, congestive heart failure or accumulation of fluid (swelling) in arms, legs, hands, or feet, kidney disease, liver disease, chronic rash such as eczema.
- Side effects: headache, nausea or decreased appetite, depression, anxiety or confusion, insomnia, nervousness, dizziness, lightheadedness, drowsiness, dry mouth, constipation.
- Close monitoring if on a diuretic.

Mondafinil (Provigil)

- Dosage: 100 mg morning (initial).
- Contraindication: angina, recent MI, cirrhosis, seizures.
- Side effects: headache, nausea, anxiety, insomnia, nervousness, dizziness.

Methylphenidate (Ritalin)

- Dosage: 5 mg morning and noon (initial).
- Contraindications: marked anxiety, tension and agitation, patients with glaucoma, seizures, motor tics, **not** in combination with a monoamine oxidase inhibitor.

- Side effects: anxiety, insomnia, nervousness, hypersensitivity reactions, anorexia, dizziness, palpitations, blood pressure alterations, cardiac arrhythmias.
- Serious adverse events reported with concomitant use with clonidine.

Bromocriptine (Parlodel)
- Dosage: 1.25 mg morning and noon (initial).
- Contraindication: uncontrolled hypertension.
- Side effects: nausea, headache, dizziness, fatigue, vomiting, drowsiness.

■ Discharge planning

Patients will either go home, to long-term acute care, to inpatient rehabilitation, to a skilled nursing facility, or to a nursing home. This should be determined after evaluating the patient's short- and long-term rehabilitation potential in conjunction with the rehabilitation team, and discussions with the patient and family over resources, home support and environment, and preferred location.

HOME

For the patient who is independent. Consider home safety evaluation, supervision level, and arrange outpatient rehabilitation services if needed.

LONG-TERM ACUTE CARE (LTAC)

For the patient who has medical needs requiring long-term hospitalization, usually for more than a month. An example would be a patient with pneumonia after a tracheostomy and PEG, or patients with other critical care or medical needs that make them too sick for an inpatient rehabilitation unit or a nursing facility because daily medical care is needed.

INPATIENT REHABILITATION

Rehabilitation completed during an inpatient stay in a rehabilitation unit of an acute care hospital, or in a free-standing rehabilitation hospital. For patients who have good rehabilitation potential but who are not yet able to function independently at home. Must be alert, cooperative, and strong enough to be able to participate in 3 hours of PT and OT daily. Medicare criteria are that patients must be able to tolerate 3 hours of therapy daily, and must require two modalities of therapy, of which one is PT. Usually lasts for 2 weeks.

SKILLED NURSING (SNF)

Rehabilitation performed during a stay in a nursing facility. For patients at a lower level than inpatient rehabilitation, these are patients who are not yet able to function independently at home, and can't participate in 3 hours of therapy daily, but do have the potential for improving to that point over the next few months. These patients must be medically stable. If needed, tracheostomy and PEG should be done before transfer. Nursing facilities vary widely in the delivery of rehabilitation services, from limited services to complete range of rehabilitation services (OT, PT, ST).

NURSING HOME

For patients who are dependent for most of their daily needs, and likely to stay that way. These patients must be medically stable. Usually a PEG does not exclude a patient, but a tracheostomy and the need for frequent suctioning means the patient will need an SNF.

Appendix 1
Numbers and calculations

Weight

1 pound = 0.4535924 kilograms
1 kilogram = 2.204622 pounds

Pressure

1 mm Hg = 1.36 cm H_2O
1 cm H_2O = 0.74 mm Hg

Mean arterial pressure (MAP)

$$\frac{SBP + (DBP \times 2)}{3}$$

Normal MAP 70–105 mm Hg

Intracranial pressure (ICP)

Normal < 10–15 mm Hg

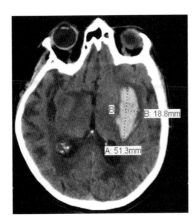

Calculating ICH volume on a CT image.
Source: J. P. Broderick, T. G. Brott, J. E. Duldner, T. Tomsick, & G. Huster, Volume of intracerebral hemorrhage: a powerful and easy-to-use predictor of 30-day mortality. *Stroke* 1993; **24**: 987–93.[83] Reproduced with permission from Lippincott Williams & Wilkins.

Cerebral perfusion pressure (CPP)

CPP = MAP – ICP
Normal CPP 70–100 mm Hg
Goal CPP > 70–80 mm Hg

Hemorrhage volume calculation

Lengths in cm:
- A and B are perpendicular diameters at the level of the largest hematoma area
- C is the thickness of the hematoma = (number of CT slices with visible hematoma) × (thickness of slice)
- Do not include intraventricular blood.

Volume in mL (cm^3) $\approx \dfrac{A \times B \times C}{2}$

Appendix 2
IV TPA dosing chart

| Patient weight | | TPA dose (mg) | | |
Pounds	Kilograms	Total	**Bolus** over 1 minute	**Infusion** over 1 hour
99 lb	**45 kg**	41	4.1	37
101 lb	46 kg	41	4.1	37
104 lb	47 kg	42	4.2	38
106 lb	48 kg	43	4.3	39
108 lb	49 kg	44	4.4	40
110 lb	**50 kg**	45	4.5	41
112 lb	51 kg	46	4.6	41
115 lb	52 kg	47	4.7	42
117 lb	53 kg	48	4.8	43
119 lb	54 kg	49	4.9	44
121 lb	55 kg	50	5.0	45
123 lb	56 kg	50	5.0	45
126 lb	57 kg	51	5.1	46
128 lb	58 kg	52	5.2	47
130 lb	59 kg	53	5.3	48
132 lb	**60 kg**	54	5.4	49
134 lb	61 kg	55	5.5	50
137 lb	62 kg	56	5.6	50
139 lb	63 kg	57	5.7	51
141 lb	64 kg	58	5.8	52
143 lb	65 kg	59	5.9	53
146 lb	66 kg	59	5.9	53
148 lb	67 kg	60	6.0	54
150 lb	68 kg	61	6.1	55
152 lb	69 kg	62	6.2	56

| Patient weight | | TPA dose (mg) | | |
Pounds	Kilograms	Total	Bolus over 1 minute	Infusion over 1 hour
154 lb	**70 kg**	63	6.3	57
157 lb	71 kg	64	6.4	58
159 lb	72 kg	65	6.5	59
161 lb	73 kg	66	6.6	59
163 lb	74 kg	67	6.7	60
165 lb	75 kg	68	6.8	61
168 lb	76 kg	68	6.8	61
170 lb	77 kg	69	6.9	62
172 lb	78 kg	70	7.0	63
174 lb	79 kg	71	7.1	64
176 lb	**80 kg**	72	7.2	65
179 lb	81 kg	73	7.3	66
181 lb	82 kg	74	7.4	67
183 lb	83 kg	75	7.5	68
185 lb	84 kg	76	7.6	68
187 lb	85 kg	77	7.7	69
190 lb	86 kg	77	7.7	69
192 lb	87 kg	78	7.8	70
194 lb	88 kg	79	7.9	71
196 lb	89 kg	80	8.0	72
198 lb	**90 kg**	81	8.1	73
201 lb	91 kg	82	8.2	74
203 lb	92 kg	83	8.3	75
205 lb	93 kg	84	8.4	76
207 lb	94 kg	85	8.5	77
209 lb	95 kg	86	8.6	77
212 lb	96 kg	86	8.6	77
214 lb	97 kg	87	8.7	78
216 lb	98 kg	88	8.8	79
218 lb	99 kg	89	8.9	80
≥220 lb	**≥100 kg**	90	9.0	81

Note:
Patients weighing more than 100 kg (220 lb) receive 90 mg (9 mg bolus and 81 mg infusion).

Appendix 3
Sample admission orders

Routine ischemic stroke

☐ STAT " PLACE **X** IN BOX IF **STAT** "

"Authorization is hereby given to dispense the Generic equivalent or Medical Staff approved therapeutic equivalent unless otherwise indicated by the words- **DO NOT SUBSTITUTE – MEDICAL NECESSITY**"

ALLERGIES: ☐ NKA ☐ YES
DRUG:_____
OTHER:_____

WT:_____kg HT:_____cm

Date	Time	PHYSICIAN'S ORDERS
		Admit to Dr._____ ☐ NTICU ☐ Stroke Unit ☐ NIMU ☐ Floor **Diagnosis:**_____ **Condition:** ☐ Stable ☐ Guarded ☐ Critical **Vitals:** ☐ Vital signs and neuro check every 1 hour × 4 hours, then q 2 hours × 8 hours, then routine ☐ Vital signs every_____hours ☐ Neuro checks every_____hours ☐ Ins and Out qshift **Call Orders:** Notify physician for the following: ☐ Change in neuro status ☐ MAP >_____mmHg or <_____(110) mmHg ☐ SBP >_____(200) mmHg or <_____mmHg ☐ DPB >_____(120) mmHg or <_____(50) mmHg ☐ Respiratory rate >_____(24) or <_____(8) ☐ Heart rate >_____(120) or <_____(50) ☐ Temperature >_____(101.4)°F or <_____°F ☐ Urinary output >_____ml/hr or <_____ml/hr **Foley catheter (MRI compatible):** ☐ Yes ☐ No ☐ Straight catheterization if unable to void **Activity:** ☐ Bed rest ☐ Up in chair_____ ☐ Head of bed 30° and initiate aspiration precautions ☐ Head of bed flat ×_____hours ☐ OOB with PT/OT ☐ Bathroom privileges with assistance **Diet:** ☐ NPO until cleared by Speech ☐ Speech consult ☐ Regular ☐ ADA_____calories ☐ Other:_____ **IV Fluids:** ☐ Saline lock ☐ **0.9NS + 20 mEq KCl/liter** @_____ml/hr ×_____L then saline lock OR call HO for further orders ☐ Other:_____ **Laboratory (if not already done):** ☐ Chem-12 ☐ Liver profile ☐ CBC with platelets ☐ Urine culture and urinalysis ☐ PT/INR/PTT ☐ Fasting lipid profile ☐ Hemoglobin A₁c ☐ Other_____
		Name_____ Print_____ Pager No./MSID #_____ Date/Time_____

Acute Ischemic Stroke Orders
(Page 1 of 2)

Please place patient sticker here

☐ **STAT** " PLACE **X** IN BOX IF **STAT** "

ALLERGIES: ☐ NKA ☐ YES
  DRUG:_____
  OTHER:_____
WT:_____ kg   HT:_____ cm

"Authorization is hereby given to dispense the Generic equivalent or Medical Staff approved therapeutic equivalent unless otherwise indicated by the words- **DO NOT SUBSTITUTE – MEDICAL NECESSITY"**

Date	Time	PHYSICIAN'S ORDERS
		Respiratory:

Under PHYSICIAN'S ORDERS:

Respiratory:
☐ O₂ per_____ at_____ l/min. Titrate Q_____hour to maintain O₂ sat ≥ _____(92)%.
☐ Check O₂ sat on room air every 8 hours; may discontinue O₂ if sat ≥ 92% on 3 readings.
☐ **Albuterol** 2.5 mg Q_____(6) hours and Q_____(2) hours PRN wheezing.
☐ **Ipratroprium bromide** 0.5 mg neb Q _____(8) hours. *Indicated in COPD.*

Diagnostic Studies:
☐ CT of head (noncontrast) @_____
☐ Exam: Brain ☐ MRI ☐ Contrast ☐ MRA
  Indication:_____
  Order Comments: ☐ Perfusion ☐ ICH protocol ☐ MRV
  Perfusion and ICH require contrast.
  List neurological sign or symptom for indication:_____
☐ Carotid doppler ultrasound
☐ CT angiogram of head and neck to include vertebral origins. Indication:_____
☐ Transcranial doppler
☐ 2-D ECHO with bubble study Indication:_____
☐ 12-lead EKG Indication:_____
☐ TEE Indication:_____

Antiplatelets:
☐ **Aspirin loading dose**_____ mg PO × 1. (Do not give if administered in ED)
☐ **Aspirin**_____ mg PO daily
☐ **Clopidogrel (Plavix)loading dose**_____ mg PO × 1. (Do not give if administered in ED)
☐ **Clopidogrel (Plavix)** 75 mg PO every day.
☐ **Dipyridamole 200mg/aspirin 25mg (Aggrenox)** 1 tablet PO every 12 hours.

Antihypertensives:
  If SBP >_____**mmHg or DBP>**_____**mmHg, give:**
☐ **Labetalol** 10– 20 mg IV over 1–2 minutes every 15 minutes × 3
  Do not give if SBP <_____mmHg or DBP < _____mmHg
  If SBP ≥ 180 or DBP ≥105 after 3 doses call physician.
☐ **Enalaprilat**_____ (0.625–1.25)mg IV over 5 minutes every 6 hours.
☐ **Other:**_____

☐ **Nicardipine** drip at ____(5) mg/hr; titrate to maintain MAP < ____(130) mmHg or SBP ≤ ____mmHg.
  Do not exceed 15 mg/hr.

Venous Thromboembolism (VTE) Prophylaxis:
☐ **SCDs and Ted Hose**
☐ **Unfractionated heparin** 5000 units SQ every_____ (12) hours. Use Q8H dosing for patients > 70 kg.*Platelet count every other day starting on Day 2*
☐ **Enoxaparin (Lovenox)** _____(30) mg SQ Q_____(12) hours. For renal impairment use 30–40 mg SQ every day. *Platelet count every other day starting on Day 2*

_____   _____   _____   _____
Name   Print   Pager No./MSID #   Date/Time

Acute Ischemic Stroke Orders
(Page 2 of 2)

Please place patient sticker here

☐ **STAT** " PLACE **X** IN BOX IF **STAT** "

"Authorization is hereby given to dispense the Generic
equivalent or Medical Staff approved therapeutic
equivalent unless otherwise indicated by the words-
DO NOT SUBSTITUTE – MEDICAL NECESSITY"

ALLERGIES: ☐ NKA ☐ YES
DRUG:_____
OTHER:_____
WT:_____ kg   HT:_____ cm

Date	Time	PHYSICIAN'S ORDERS

Blood Glucose Therapy:

☐ FSBG every 4 hours.   Administer **Regular** human insulin SQ.

Blood Glucose	
≤60 mg/dl	Repeat FSBG; If < 60 mg/dl, give 50 ml D_{50}W IV and call HO, repeat FSBG in 15 minutes
61–110 mg/dl	Do not administer insulin
111–125 mg/dl	3 units
126–150 mg/dl	5 units
>150 mg/dl	7 units, call HO for 2 consecutive FSBG > 150 mg/dl

Laxative Therapy:
☐ Docusate sodium 100 mg PO every 12 hours.
☐ Bisacodyl 10 mg suppository PR every day PRN.
☐ Milk of Magnesia 30–60 m lPO PRN if no results from bisacodyl.

Stress Ulcer Prophylaxis:
☐ **Famotidine** (Pepcid) 20 mg PO <u>OR</u> IV every 12 hours. *Circle route.*

Analgesic/Antipyretic Therapy:
☐ **Acetaminophen** 650 mg PO <u>OR</u> PR every 4 hours PRN temperature greater than 101.5° F *Circle route.*
☐ Cooling blanket

Rehabilitation:
☐ Stroke Rehab (*advise patients with ongoing neurological deficits*)
☐ Physical therapy
☐ Occupational therapy
☐ Nutrition consult
☐ Speech therapy
☐ Chaplain consult
☐ PM&R

Discharge Planning:
☐ Financial Counselor consult

Other Orders:

_____

_____

_____

Name	Print	Pager No./MSID #	Date/Time

Post-TPA

☐ STAT " PLACE **X** IN BOX IF **STAT** "

"Authorization is hereby given to dispense the Generic equivalent or Medical Staff approved therapeutic equivalent unless otherwise indicated by the words- **DO NOT SUBSTITUTE – MEDICAL NECESSITY"**

ALLERGIES: ☐ NKA ☐ YES
DRUG:_____
OTHER:_____

WT:_____ kg   HT:_____ cm

Date	Time	PHYSICIAN'S ORDERS

		Admit to Dr._____
		   ☐ NTICU ☐ Stroke Unit ☐ NIMU ☐ Floor
		
		 Diagnosis:_____
		 Condition: ☐ Stable ☐ Guarded ☐ Critical
		
		 Vitals:
		   ☐ Vital signs and neuro check every 1 hour × 4 hours, then q 2 hours × 8 hours, then routine
		   ☐ Monitor BP q15 minutes × 2 hours, q30 minutes × 6 hours, then q1hour × 16 hours
		   ☐ Telemetry × 24 hours
		   ☐ Neuro checks every_____ hours
		   ☐ Ins and Out qshift
		
		 Call Orders:
		 Notify physician for the following:
		   ☐ Change in neuro status
		   ☐ Angioedema
		   ☐ Signs and symptoms of bleeding
		   ☐ MAP >_____mmHg or <_____ (110) mmHg
		   ☐ SBP >_____ (180) mmHg or <_____mmHg
		   ☐ DPB >_____ (105) mmHg or <_____ (50) mmHg
		   ☐ Respiratory rate >_____(24) or <_____(8)
		   ☐ Heart rate >_____(120) or <_____(50)
		   ☐ Temperature >_____(101.4)°F or <_____°F
		   ☐ Urinary output >_____ml/hr or <_____ml/hr
		
		 Foley catheter (MRI compatible): ☐ Yes ☐ No ☐ Straight catheterization if unable to void
		
		 Activity:
		   ☐ Bed rest × 24 hours except for PT,OT, Rehab evaluation
		   ☐ Head of bed flat × 12 hours
		   ☐ Avoid arterial sticks and other procedures that may increase risk of bleeding × 24 hours
		
		 Diet:
		   ☐ NPO until cleared by Speech
		   ☐ Speech consult
		   ☐ Regular ☐ ADA_____calories ☐ Other:_____
		
		 IV Fluids:
		   ☐ Saline lock
		   ☐ **0.9NS + 20 mEq KCl/liter** @ _____ml/hr × ____L then saline lock <u>OR</u> call HO for further orders
		   ☐ Other:_____
		
		 Laboratory (if not already done):
		   ☐ Chem-12
		   ☐ CBC with differential and platelets
		   ☐ Urine culture and urinalysis
		   ☐ PT/INR/PTT
		   ☐ Fasting lipid profile
		   ☐ Hemoglobin A_{1c}
		   ☐ Liver profile ☐ Other:_____

Name	Print	Pager No./MSID # Date/Time

Acute Ischemic Stroke Orders:
Post t-PA
(Page 1 of 2)

Please place patient sticker here

☐ **STAT** " PLACE **X** IN BOX IF **STAT** "

ALLERGIES: ☐ NKA ☐ YES
DRUG: _____
OTHER: _____
WT: _____ kg HT: _____ cm

"Authorization is hereby given to dispense the Generic equivalent or Medical Staff approved therapeutic equivalent unless otherwise indicated by the words-
DO NOT SUBSTITUTE – MEDICAL NECESSITY"

Date	Time	PHYSICIAN'S ORDERS
		Respiratory: ☐ O₂ per_____at _____l/min. Titrate Q_____hour to maintain O₂ sat ≥ _____(92)%. ☐ Check O₂ sat on room air every 8 hours; may discontinue O₂ if sat ≥ 92% on 3 readings. ☐ **Albuterol** 2.5 mg Q _____(6) hours and Q _____(2) hours PRN wheezing. ☐ **Ipratropium bromide** 0.5 mg neb Q _____(8) hours. *Indicated for COPD.* **Diagnostic Studies:** ☐ CT of head (noncontrast) @ _____ ☐ Exam: Brain ☐ MRI ☐ Contrast ☐ MRA Indication:_____ Order Comments: ☐ Perfusion ☐ ICH protocol ☐ MRV *Perfusion and ICH require contrast.* *List neurological sign or symptom for indication:*_____ ☐ Carotid doppler ultrasound ☐ CT angiogram of head and neck to include vertebral origins. Indication:_____ ☐ Transcranial doppler ☐ 2-D ECHO with bubble study Indication:_____ ☐ 12-lead EKG Indication:_____ ☐ TEE Indication:_____ **Antihypertensives:** **If SBP >_____mmHg or DBP>_____mmHg, give:** ☐ **Labetalol** 10–20 mg IV over 1–2 minutes every 15 minutes × 3 *Do not give if SBP <_____mmHg or DBP <_____mmHg* *If SBP ≥ 180 or DBP ≥ 105 after 3 doses call physician.* ☐ **Enalaprilat**_____ (0.625 – 1.25)mg IV over 5 minutes every 6 hours. ☐ Other:_____ ☐ **Nicardipine** drip at ____(5) mg/hr; titrate to maintain MAP < ____(110) mmHg or SBP ≤ _____mmHg. *Do not exceed 15 mg/hr.* **Venous Thromboembolism (VTE) Prophylaxis:** ☐ SCDs and Ted Hose NO aspirin, plavix, aggrenox, coumadin or heparin × 24 hours
		Name _____ Print _____ Pager No./MSID # _____ Date/Time _____

Acute Ischemic Stroke Orders:
Post t-PA
(Page 2 of 2)

Please place patient sticker here

☐ **STAT** " PLACE **X** IN BOX IF **STAT** "

"Authorization is hereby given to dispense the Generic equivalent or Medical Staff approved therapeutic quivalent unless otherwise indicated by the words-
DO NOT SUBSTITUTE – MEDICAL NECESSITY"

ALLERGIES: ☐ NKA ☐ YES
DRUG:_____
OTHER:_____
W I:_____ kg HT:_____ cm

Date	Time	PHYSICIAN'S ORDERS

Blood Glucose Therapy:

☐ FSBG every 4 hours. Administer **Regular** human insulin SQ.

Blood Glucose	
≤60 mg/dl	Repeat FSBG; If < 60 mg/dl, give 50 ml D_{50}W IV and call HO, repeat FSBG in 15 minutes
61–110 mg/dl	Do not administer insulin
111–125 mg/dl	3 units
126–150 mg/dl	5 units
>150 mg/dl	7 units, call HO for 2 consecutive FSBG > 150 mg/dl

Laxative Therapy:
☐ Docusate sodium 100 mg PO every 12 hours.
☐ Bisacodyl 10 mg suppository PR every day PRN.
☐ Milk of Magnesia 30–60 ml PO PRN if no results from bisacodyl.

Stress Ulcer Prophylaxis:
☐ **Famotidine** (Pepcid) 20 mg PO <u>OR</u> IV every 12 hours. *Circle route.*

Analgesic/Antipyretic Therapy:
☐ **Acetaminophen** 650 mg PO <u>OR</u> PR every 4 hours PRN temperature greater than 101.5 °F *Circle route.*
☐ Cooling blanket

Rehabilitation:
☐ Stroke Rehab (*advise patients with ongoing neurological deficits*)
☐ Physical therapy
☐ Occupational therapy
☐ Nutrition consult
☐ Speech therapy
☐ Chaplain consult
☐ PM&R

Discharge Planning:
☐ Financial Counselor consult

Other Orders:

_____

_____

_____

Name	Print	Pager No./MSID #	Date/Time

Appendix 4
Sample discharge summary

Name

Medical record number

Admitting date, service, and attending physician

Discharge date, service, and attending physician (if different from admission)

Discharge diagnosis

Be specific regarding type and cause of stroke, and include risk factors and other important diagnoses, e.g.

(1) cardioembolic ischemic stroke

(2) atrial fibrillation

(3) hypertension

History of present illness

- Presenting symptoms (be specific, including time of onset)
- Past medical history
- Past surgical history
- Medications on admission
- Relevant social history
- Relevant family history
- Relevant review of systems

- Physical exam
  - Include general exam as well as neurologic exam
  - Include NIH stroke scale if possible
- Labs
- Radiology
- Procedures
- Consults

Hospital course

- Include acute treatment, diagnostic work-up, neurologic course, complications
- Stroke mechanism
  - For **ischemia**: cardioembolic, carotid stenosis, intracranial stenosis, lacunar stroke, dissection, venous, cryptogenic, etc.
  - For **ICH**: hypertensive, AVM, amyloid angiopathy, unknown, etc.
- Condition at discharge: stable, etc.
  - Also describe remaining deficits, impairment
  - Discharge NIH stroke scale
- Disposition: home, skilled nursing facility, inpatient rehabilitation, etc.
- Discharge medications
- Instructions to patients
  - Physical activity
  - Diet
  - Smoking cessation counseling, etc.
  - Follow-up plan

Send copy to primary care provider.

Appendix 5
Stroke radiology

COMPUTED TOMOGRAPHY (CT)

Non-contrast head CT remains the standard procedure for
initial evaluation of stroke.

Acute ischemia appearances (general guidelines)

- <6 hours: no change in appearance, or
- >1.5 hours: loss of grey–white differentiation
- >3 hours: hypodensity
- >6 hours: swelling
- >weeks: ex-vacuo changes

Window width and level (WW/WL) for early CT

The standard brain view on CT is set at around 90/40. Setting of
$\sim$25/$\sim$30 may give high contrast of brain parenchyma to
demonstrate the early ischemic signs more easily.

Acute hemorrhage (extravasated blood)

Appears hyperdense (bright) in 40–60 Hounsefield units
(HU). In the first few hours, the intensity may increase to
60–80 HUs. Intensity attenuates with time at a rate of
$\sim$0.7–1.5 HU/day.

The role of contrast head CT

CT angiography

- Involves IV bolus of contrast, and imaging the arteries quickly during first pass of contrast.
- Allows visualization of vessels or lack thereof (occlusion, stenosis, AVM, aneurysms).
- Requirements:
  - adequate renal function because the contrast bolus is more than usual;
  - good IV access (you don't want contrast in soft tissues!).
- CT viewing window width/level at 800/100 may be best to visualize the arteries next to bones.

Standard contrast head CT

- Allows evaluation for stroke mimics by detecting blood–brain barrier breakdown:
  - Tumor, infection, inflammation, etc.

How to try to prevent contrast nephropathy

- **Acetylcysteine** 600 mg PO every 12 hours the day before and the day of iodinated contrast administration for CT or angiography.[98,99]
- **Sodium bicarbonate**:[100]
  - 154 mEq/L of sodium bicarbonate in dextrose and H_2O (adding 154 mL of 1000 mEq/L sodium bicarbonate to 846 mL of 5% dextrose);
  - IV bolus at 3 mL/kg per hour × 1 hour immediately before radiocontrast injection (maximum 330 mL/hr);
  - followed by 1 mL/kg per hour during the contrast exposure and for 6 hours after the procedure (maximum 110 mL/hr).

- Adequate hydration.
- Creatinine >2.0 probably contraindicates use of IV contrast in most cases.

ASPECTS (Alberta Stroke Programme Early CT Score)

ASPECTS is a reliable scoring system of early CT changes in MCA territory infarction in the first few hours of ischemic stroke.[101] Non-contrast CT scans are interpreted at two levels:

(a) at the level of basal ganglia and thalamus.
(b) at the level just rostral to basal ganglia.

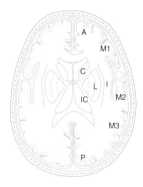

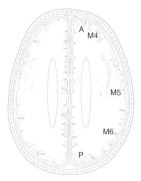

(a) at the level of basal ganglia and thalamus

(b) at the level just rostral to basal ganglia

ASPECTS template.

Source: P. A. Barber, A. M. Demchuk, J. Zhang, & A. M. Buchan, Validity and reliability of a quantitative computed tomography score in predicting outcome of hyperacute stroke before thrombolytic therapy. ASPECTS Study Group. Alberta Stroke Programme Early CT Score. *Lancet* 2000; **355**: 1670–4.[101] Copyright © 1974, with permission from Elsevier.

ASPECTS study form

	10 regions of interest
At the level of basal ganglia and thalamus	At the level just rostral to basal ganglia
C = caudate	
L = lentiform nuclei	
IC = internal capsule	
I = insular cortex	
M1 = anterior MCA cortex	M4 (superior to M1)
M2 = MCA cortex lateral to insula	M5 (superior to M2)
M3 = posterior MCA cortex	M6 (superior to M3)

Notes:

(Not included in scoring: A = ACA circulation; P = PCA circulation)

Subcortical structures are allotted 3 points (C, L, and IC).

MCA cortex is allotted 7 points (insular cortex, M1, M2, M3, M4, M5, and M6).

1 point is subtracted for each defined area of early ischemic change, such as **focal swelling**, or **parenchymal hypoattenuation**. The score varies from 10 to 0:

- 10 = normal.
- 0 = abnormal in entire MCA distribution.

MAGNETIC RESONANCE IMAGING (MRI)

You have to refer to a real MRI book to explain all the physics of the sequences. Here is a brief simplification of what each one looks like and what they are used for.

T1-weighted sequence (usually in axial and sagittal sections)

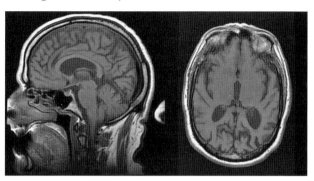

How to identify
- Usually looks pale and bland. It looks the "most similar to CT." It appears exactly how you would expect the brain to look: cerebrospinal fluid is black; gray matter is gray; white matter is white.

Use
- Good for anatomy.
- Compare to T1 with contrast for leakage of blood–brain barrier.

T2-weighted sequence

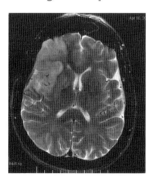

How to identify
- Exactly the opposite of how you would expect the brain to look: cerebrospinal fluid is white; gray matter is light; white matter is dark.

Use
- Good for pathology, and to evaluate flow voids.
- White: cerebrospinal fluid, edema, ischemia, and most bad things.
- Dark: old blood.

FLAIR (fluid-attenuated inversion recovery)

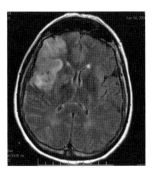

How to identify
- Cerebrospinal fluid is dark; gray matter is light; white matter is dark.
- It is essentially T2 with CSF made black.

Use
- Same as T2. It makes it easy to find pathology at CSF/brain junction (multiple sclerosis plaques, metastases, etc.) since on T2 it is sometimes difficult to tell what is CSF and what is pathological tissue.

- White: edema, ischemia, and most bad things.
- Dark: CSF, old blood.

Tips for identifying T1, T2 and FLAIR images

(1) Look at CSF:
  - (a) If it is white, it is T2.
  - (b) If it is dark, go to step 2.
(2) Look at gray and white matter:
  - (a) If it is normal, it is T1.
  - (b) If it is reversed, it is a FLAIR.

DWI (diffusion-weighted imaging)

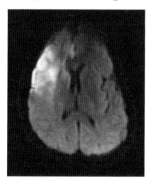

How to identify
- Uniformly gray grainy image.

Use
- Shows acute ischemia.
- White: acute ischemia (the proper term is restricted diffusion).
- Gray: everything else.

- With acute ischemic stroke, Na/K ATPase fails and cells swell. Intracellular H_2O is less mobile than H_2O in extracellular matrix. DWI is derived from the proton of the hydrogen atom.

Caution

- "T2 shine-through" – acute ischemia should be bright on DWI, dark on ADC (see below). Sometimes when T2 white-ness is strong in an old stroke, it "shines through" into DWI sequences. That's not acute stroke.
- Artifacts at air/bone interfaces – usually occur next to tem-poral bone and sinuses. These artifacts are usually symmetric and can be identified.
- Things not stroke – it turns out that many non-stroke things can appear bright on DWI. So look carefully for T2 shine-through and think whether the pattern is stroke-like (arterial distribution). Creutzfeldt–Jakob disease has cortical ribbons of DWI brightness. Wernicke's encephalopathy shows restricted DWI symmetrically around the aqueduct and in mammillary bodies.
- DWI usually indicates irreversible ischemic damage, but in the first few hours, especially if not densely white (i.e., ADC not very low), DWI abnormalities can be reversed by reperfusion.

Time course of DWI intensity

- Maximal at 40 hours.
- Normalizes in 2 to several weeks.[102]

ADC (apparent diffusion coefficient)

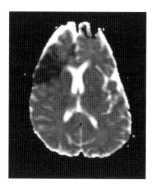

How to identify
- Grainy image with cerebrospinal fluid white.

Use
- Companion to DWI interpretation of acute ischemia.
- Dark on ADC in area where DWI is bright (white) is ischemia.
- One can think of it as "raw data" on DWI, except that ischemia is black. One can obtain quantitative measurements in the reduction in diffusion coefficient.

Time course
- Maximal (dark) at 28 hours.
- Pseudonormalizes at 10 days, then bright.[102]

MPGR (gradient-echo sequence)

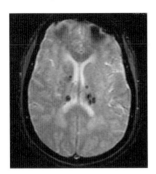

How to identify
- Grayish (it's hard by just looking).

Use
- Hemorrhages, whether new or old, appear dark.
- It is useful when looking for micro-hemorrhages such as those from amyloid angiopathy and cavernous malformations.
- One cannot measure the size of the hematoma on this image since the signal is amplified and is bigger than the amount of blood.

PWI (perfusion-weighted imaging)

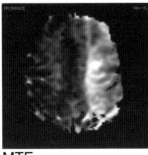 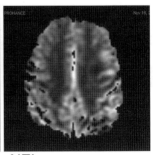

MTE   NEI

How to identify

There are two different sequences used:

- Mean time to enhancement (MTE) measures arrival time of bolus of dye. Areas of low cerebral perfusion look brighter (more light gray).
- Negative enhancement integral (NEI) measures cerebral blood volume (CBV). Areas of severe ischemia have reduced CBV and look dark. In mild ischemia, the vascular bed is dilated, CBV may be increased, and such regions will look bright.

Use

- PWI sequences measure cerebral blood flow.
- Look for a so-called "**mismatch**" between the changes on DWI, which are generally considered irreversible (but see fourth **Caution** under DWI), and areas where there is a perfusion deficit on PWI. The areas of mismatch represent tissue at risk of infarction.

MRA (magnetic resonance angiography)

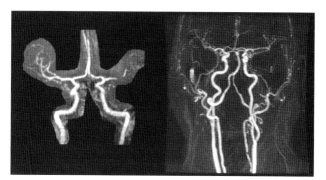

How to identify

• You see the vessels.

Use

• Arterial stenosis: signal dropout more specific than appearance of stenosis.
• Aneurysms, vascular malformations (mostly AVM).

Caution

There are a lot of artifacts in MRA images.

• It's an artifact if there are consistent findings throughout a slice (e.g., image shifted).
• It shows flow rather than artery size. Therefore in patent but low flow states, MRA may falsely give the impression of occlusion.
• Some MRA sequences are flow-direction sensitive. Reversed flow may appear as absent flow.
• MRA tends to overestimate stenosis.

Ask a well-trained person to help with interpretation.

If you are really interested in extracranial anatomy, especially aortic arch and vertebral origins, order MRA with contrast and speak to MRI technicians to insure they know what you want.

MRV (magnetic resonance venography)

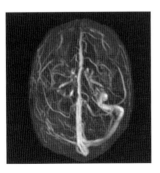

How to identify
- You see the veins.

Use
- Suspected venous sinus thrombosis. Suspect if hemorrhagic infarct, especially if bilateral, located high in convexity, associated with more edema than usual, or not fitting the usual arterial distribution of infarcts.

Caution
- Venous anatomy is variable. Especially troublesome is normal asymmetry of transverse sinuses. Ask for help in interpretation.

Usual sequences ordered for acute ischemic stroke patients

Estimated time 40 minutes.
- Sagittal T1
- Axial DWI
- Axial ADC
- Axial T1
- Axial FLAIR
- Axial MPGR
- PWI (MTE and NEI)
- Axial T1 post-contrast (if PWI is done)
- Coronal T1 post-contrast (if PWI is done)
- MRA circle of Willis and neck

MRI findings in hemorrhage

Sequential signal intensity (SI) changes of intracranial hemorrhage on MRI (1.5 T)					
	Hyperacute hemorrhage	Acute hemorrhage	Early subacute hemorrhage	Late subacute hemorrhage	Chronic hemorrhage
What happens	Blood leaves the vascular system (extravasation)	Deoxygenation with formation of deoxy-Hb	Clot retraction and deoxy-Hb is oxidized to met-Hb	Cell lysis (membrane disruption)	Macrophages digest the clot
Time frame	<12 h	Hours to days (weeks in center of hematoma)	A few days	4–7 days to 1 month	Weeks to years
Red blood cells	Intact erythrocytes	Intact, but hypoxic erythrocytes	Still intact, severely hypoxic	Lysis (solution of lysed cells)	Gone; encephalomalacia with proteinaceous fluid

Sequential signal (cont.)

	Hyperacute hemorrhage	Acute hemorrhage	Early subacute hemorrhage	Late subacute hemorrhage	Chronic hemorrhage
State of Hb	Intracellular oxy-Hb	Intracellular deoxy-Hb	Intracellular met-Hb (first at periphery of clot)	Extracellular met-Hb	Hemosiderin (insoluble) and ferritin (water soluble)
T1-weighted images	$\approx$ or $\downarrow$	$\approx$ (or $\downarrow$)	$\uparrow\uparrow$	$\uparrow\uparrow$	$\approx$ or $\downarrow$
T2-weighted images	$\uparrow$ (High water content)	$\downarrow$ T2 PRE (susceptibility effect)	$\downarrow\downarrow$ T2 PRE (susceptibility effect)	$\uparrow\uparrow$ No T2 PRE (loss of compartmentalization)	$\downarrow\downarrow$ T2 PRE (susceptibility effect)

Notes:

Hb, hemoglobin; e-, electrons; T2 PRE, T2-proton relaxation enhancement; $\approx$, isointense relative to normal gray matter; $\uparrow$, increased SI relative to normal gray matter; $\downarrow$, decreased SI relative to normal gray matter; $\downarrow\downarrow$, markedly decreased SI relative to normal gray matter.

Source: Adapted from: P. M. Parizel, S. Makkat, E. Van Miert, J. W. Van Goethem, L. van den Hauwe, & A. M. De Schepper, Intracranial hemorrhage: principles of CT and MRI interpretation. *Eur. Radiol.* 2001; **11**: 1770–83.[103] Reproduced with kind permission from Springer Science and Business Media.

Abbreviated protocol for uncooperative patients

Estimated time 10 minutes.

- DWI
- MRA circle of Willis and neck
- T2 or FLAIR

Usual sequences ordered for acute ICH patients

- Sagittal T1
- Axial T1
- Axial T2
- Axial FLAIR
- Axial MPGR
- Axial T1 post-contrast
- Coronal T1 post-contrast
- MRA circle of Willis
- MR venography can be considered

Appendix 6
Transcranial Doppler ultrasound (TCD)

For various uses of TCD in stroke refer to Alexandrov, *Cerebrovascular Ultrasound in Stroke Prevention and Treatment* (2004).[104]

There are many uses of TCD:

- Diagnosis of intracranial stenosis
- Diagnosis of acute occlusion
- Monitoring of acute thrombolytic therapy
- Vasoreactivity (vascular reserve) with carotid disease
- Emboli monitoring
- Vascular monitoring during surgery
- Detection of right-to-left shunt (RLS) (most commonly patent foramen ovale)

Procedure for right-to-left shunt detection

Based on European Society of Neurosonology and Cerebral Hemodynamics consensus, 1999.[105,106]

Equipment

- TCD
- two normal saline bottles 15 cm^3
- two 10 cm^3 syringes
- flexible tubing
- three-way stopcock

Preparation

- The patient must be in the supine position, with the arm horizontal. An intravenous catheter (#18) is inserted into an antecubital vein (connected to a 250 ml bottle of physiologic solution by means of a flexible tube to maintain venous access).
- The right middle cerebral artery is traced by means of TCD (the examination is more sensitive if bilateral monitoring is used).

Procedure

- Two 10 ml (or 20 ml) syringes are prepared: one containing 9 ml of physiologic solution and the other containing 1 ml of air. By means of a three-way stopcock, the contents of both syringes are rapidly mixed until a homogeneous solution is obtained.
- The solution is rapidly injected in bolus form with the patient at rest. Inject with the syringe pointed superiorly so the bubbles aggregate at the top and are injected first.
- The MCA is monitored for 40–60 seconds.

The procedure is repeated with Valsalva maneuver

- The efficacy of the Valsalva maneuver must be ascertained beforehand through the reduction of the systolic flow velocity on MCA by at least one-third.
- Five seconds after injection of the contrast agent, the examiner orders the patient to begin the Valsalva maneuver, which must last for at least 10 seconds.

Interpretation

The test is deemed positive if the appearance of at least one microbubble (MB) is recorded as high-intensity transient signal (HITS) on the TCD trace within 40 seconds of terminating the injection; no agreement exists as to a cutoff interval between contrast injection and microbubble appearance.

Although it takes about 11 seconds for the bubbles to reach the MCA through an intracardiac shunt, and about 14 seconds through an intrapulmonary shunt, a time window cannot differentiate between RLS at the atrial level and RLS at different sites of the vascular system. It is in any case advisable to record the time of appearance of the first MB.

The results of the two sessions (basal and with Valsalva) must be evaluated separately. Repeated testing may increase the sensitivity, and in the event of discrepancies the positive test must be considered.

- No HITS: **test negative**.
- 1–10 HITS: **low-grade shunt**.
- >10 HITS, but without "curtain" effect: **medium-grade shunt**.

- Curtain effect, seen when the microbubbles are so numerous as to be no longer distinguishable separately: **high-grade shunt**.

With regard to the physiopathological features of the RLS, we define as:

- Permanent – a shunt detected in basal conditions.
- Latent – a shunt detected only with Valsalva.

Appendix 7
Heparin protocol

Modified from Toth and Voll, 2002.[107]

- Check hematocrit, platelet count, INR, PTT at baseline (within the prior 72 hours).
- Obtain or estimate patient's weight (use **adjusted body weight** for obese patients).
- **No bolus heparin**.

Initial heparin infusion	
Weight	Initial infusion
<50 kg	500 units/hr = 10 ml/hr
50–59 kg	600 units/hr = 12 ml/hr
60–69 kg	700 units/hr = 14 ml/hr
70–79 kg	800 units/hr = 16 ml/hr
80–89 kg	900 units/hr = 18 ml/hr
90–99 kg	1000 units/hr = 20 ml/hr
100–109 kg	1100 units/hr = 22 ml/hr
110–119 kg	1200 units/hr = 24 ml/hr
>119 kg	1400 units/hr = 28 ml/hr

- Check PTT every 6 hours after change in infusion or every 24 hours if within therapeutic range.
- CBC every 3 days.
- Goal PTT 55–85 seconds.

- Adjustment every 6 hours.
- Check platelet count daily. A 50% decrease may indicate heparin-induced thrombocytopenia (see Appendix 9).

Heparin infusion adjustment

PTT (sec)	Stop infusion	Change rate of infusion	Check PTT
<45		↑ 200 units/hr	in 6 hours
45–54		↑ 100 units/hr	in 6 hours
55–85		No change	in 6 hours
86–90		↓ 100 units/hr	next morning
91–100	30 minutes	↓ 150 units/hr	in 6 hours
>100	60 minutes	↓ 250 units/hr	in 6 hours

- Call physician if PTT < 45 or > 100 seconds on two consecutive measurements, or if > 125 seconds.
- If significant bleeding occurs, stop heparin and assess.

Appendix 8
Insulin protocol

Insulin drip

Make sure that the nursing unit is capable of using insulin drip with glucose measurement every 1 hour.

- Use insulin drip if the glucose in an acute stroke patient is over 250 mg/dL.
- Target insulin level 80–110 mg/dL.
  - Check capillary glucose every 1 hour.
  - Consider insulin bolus.
  - Start insulin drip at the calculated rate using the following formula:

    (blood sugar – 60) $\times$ 0.03 $\rightarrow$ __units/hr IV drip.

  - Readjust glucose infusion every 1 hour using the above formula.
  - If glucose is <200, then do glucose check every 2 hours.
  - If glucose is <60, give 1 ampoule D50 and call physician.

Regular insulin sliding scale

Recommended indications

- As a **supplement** to a patient's usual diabetes medications (long-acting insulin or oral agents) to treat uncontrolled high blood sugars.

- For short-term use (24–48 hours) in a patient admitted with an unknown insulin requirement.

Regimens: insulin sliding-scale protocol

Blood sugar (mg/dL)	Low-dose scale	Moderate-dose scale	High-dose scale	Patient-specific scale
<60	Initiate hypoglycemia protocol	Initiate hypoglycemia protocol	Initiate hypoglycemia protocol	Initiate hypoglycemia protocol
60–130	0 units	0 units	0 units	__ units
131–180	2 units	4 units	8 units	__ units
181–240	4 units	8 units	12 units	__ units
241–300	6 units	10 units	16 units	__ units
301–350	8 units	12 units	20 units	__ units
351–400	10 units	16 units	24 units	__ units
>400	12 units and call physician	20 units and call physician	28 units and call physician	__ units

Notes:
Low-dose scale: suggested starting point for thin and elderly, or those being initiated on total parenteral nutrition.
Moderate-dose scale: suggested starting point for average patient.
High-dose scale: suggested for patients with infections or those receiving therapy with high-dose corticosteroids.

Check blood sugars
- Before meals and at bedtime (06:30, 11:30, 16:30, 21:30 h).
- Twice daily (06:30, 16:30 h).
- Every 6 hours (recommended for patients receiving continuous nutrition over 24 hours).
- Every 4 hours (recommended for patients requiring close monitoring).

Appendix 9
Medical complications

This appendix deals with the prevention and treatment of **deep venous thrombosis**, **aspiration pneumonia**, **urinary tract infection**, and **heparin-induced thrombocytopenia**.

All of these are common complications in stroke patients. Heparin-induced thrombocytopenia, while not common, is under-diagnosed.

Deep venous thrombosis (DVT)

Prevention
- Enoxaparin (Lovenox) 40 mg SC once daily: probably the best choice.[108]
  - In very large patients, consider 30 mg SC every 12 hours.
- Heparin 5000 units SC every 12 hours.*
- Dalteparin (Fragmin) 5000 units once daily.
- Compressive stockings and sequential compression devices (SCDs).

Diagnosis
- Leg vein Doppler ultrasound sometimes confirmed by X-ray or MRI venography.

Treatment
- Full dose weight-adjusted heparin (see Appendix 7).

Aspiration pneumonia

Prevention
- NPO until speech pathology evaluation or bedside evaluation by specially trained nurses.
- Follow speech pathology recommendations.
- Head of bed up.
- Sit upright when eating.
- Assistance with feeding.

Diagnosis
A constellation of symptoms and signs:
- fever, hypoxia, chest X-ray infiltrate, leukocytosis, clinical aspiration;
- sputum culture not very reliable.

Treatment
- No need to cover for anaerobes.
- Cover for Gram+ and Gram− (Pseudomonas, Enterobacteraciae).

Antibiotic choices
Be sure to check the patient's allergies.
- Ceftriaxone (Rocephin) 1–2 grams IV once daily.
- Cefepime (Maxipime) 1 gram IV every 12 hours.
- Gatifloxacin (Tequin) 400 mg IV/PO once daily.

- For MRSA: vancomycin (Vancocin) 1 gram IV every 12 hours (check trough levels before third or fourth dose. Target 10–20 µg/ml).
- For MSSA: nafcillin (Nallpen) 0.5–2 gram every 4 hours is better. Cefepime has fair coverage.

Duration 10–14 days.

Catheter-associated urinary tract infection (UTI)

Prevention

Remove indwelling catheter as soon as possible!

Diagnosis

- White blood cells in urinalysis.
- Urine culture of single species $> 10^5$.

Treatment

Remove or change catheter *and* a choice of

- Trimethoprim-sulfamethoxazole double strength (TMP-SMX, Bactrim DS) 1 tablet PO every 12 hours
  or
- TMP-SMX suspension 20 cc per nasojejunal (NJ) tube every 12 hours
  - Interaction: increases warfarin effect!
- Nitrofurantoin (Furadantin, Macrodantin) 50 mg capsule or suspension PO or per NJ tube every 6 hours
- Nitrofurantoin SR (Macrobid) 100 mg capsule PO every 12 hours
- Gatifloxacin 200 mg IV/PO once daily (for very ill, allergies)

Duration 3–5 days.

Check culture for final antibiotic choice.

Heparin-induced thrombocytopenia (HIT)

Prevention
Don't use heparin unless necessary, and check platelet counts daily.

Diagnosis
HIT is **underdiagnosed**. 50% of patients given unfractionated heparin develop antibodies and 3% get HIT with thrombotic syndrome (HITTS). It is more common with intravenous vs. subcutaneous use, high dose vs. low dose, unfractionated vs. low molecular weight (rare).

- Platelets drop 50% compared with baseline or <100 000. **Check platelet count daily in patients on heparin**. Check PF4 antiplatelet antibodies.
- Clinical consequences include DVT, pulmonary emboli, cardioembolism, peripheral vascular occlusion, MI, stroke.
- Consider HITTS in any patient with unexplained thrombo-embolic event post heparin exposure. Remember, platelet count may not be low – just 50% drop compared with base-line, and baseline may be well above 200 000.
- Type 1: transient, mild, starts 4 days after exposure but can start after a longer interval and after heparin is stopped.
- Type 2: two types:
  - 4–14 days after exposure.
  - <12 hours after exposure.

Treatment
Stop heparin.
Even so, 50% will still develop HITTS once platelet count starts to fall if you just stop heparin.

- Thrombin inhibitor even before platelet antibody test result is back.
  - Argatroban: reversible, more potent, non-antigenic, hepatic clearance. Half life $= 40$–50 min, adjust PTT every 2–4 hours to 1.5–3 $\times$ control. Start at 2 μg/min; titrate up to <10 μg/min.
  - Lepirudin (Refludan): irreversible, antigenic, renal clearance. Bolus 0.4 mg/kg then infusion.
- No warfarin until platelets normalize.
- No platelets.

Appendix 10
Brainstem syndromes

The pattern of cranial nerve abnormalities is the key to distinguishing among these.

Lateral medullary syndrome

Also known as **Wallenberg syndrome**. The crossed sensory findings, i.e., loss of sensation on one side of the face and the other side of the body, are pathognomonic.

- vertigo, nausea, diplopia
- ipsilateral headache (descending spinal tract of the fifth cranial nerve, facial or eye pain)
- ataxia, hiccups
- contralateral body hemianalgesia (pain + temperature)
- ipsilateral facial hemianalgesia (pain + temperature)
- Horner's syndrome, nystagmus
- ipsilateral palate, vocal cord weakness (nucleus ambiguus)
- dysphagia
- cerebellar findings
- motor, tongue function, dorsal column function spared because these structures lie medially in the medulla
- due to occlusion of the ipsilateral vertebral artery or its major branch, the posterior inferior cerebellar artery

Millard–Gubler syndrome

Ventrocaudal pons with CN VI and VII involvement
- contralateral hemiplegia (pyramidal tract)
- ipsilateral lateral rectus paresis (VI)
- ipsilateral lower motor neuron (LMN) facial paresis (VII)

Foville syndrome

Dorsal caudal pontine lesion
- contralateral body hemiplegia
- ipsilateral LMN facial paresis (VII)
- inability to move eyes to same side as lesion (parapontine reticular formation, CN VI)

Raymond–Cestan syndrome

Dorsal rostral pons
- ataxia with coarse tremor
- contralateral hemisensory loss (face + body, all modalities)
- +/− contralateral hemiparesis

Marie–Foix syndrome

Lateral pons
- ipsilateral cerebellar ataxia
- contralateral hemiparesis
- +/− contralateral hemisensory loss (pain and temperature) due to spinothalamic tract

Weber syndrome

Ventral midbrain
- contralateral hemiplegia (corticospinal and corticobulbar tracts)
- ipsilateral oculomotor paresis, dilated pupil

Benedikt syndrome

Midbrain tegmentum (red nucleus, CN III)
- ipsilateral oculomotor paresis, dilated pupil
- contralateral intention tremor, hemichorea, hemiathetosis

Claude's syndrome

Midbrain tegmentum
- ipsilateral oculomotor paresis
- contralateral cerebellar ataxia

Parinaud's syndrome

Dorsal midbrain (often with hydrocephalus, tumor)
- upgaze paresis
- convergence-retraction nystagmus on upgaze
- large pupil with light-near dissociation, lid retraction, lid lag

Appendix 11
Cerebral arterial anatomy

Circle of Willis

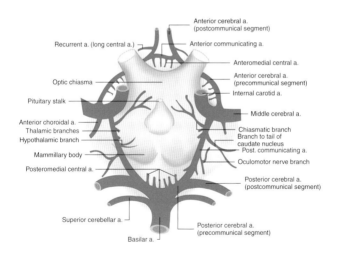

Anterior cerebral a. (postcommunical segment)

Recurrent a. (long central a.)

Anterior communicating a.

Anteromedial central a.

Optic chiasma

Anterior cerebral a. (precommunical segment)

Internal carotid a.

Pituitary stalk

Middle cerebral a.

Anterior choroidal a.
Thalamic branches
Hypothalamic branch

Chiasmatic branch
Branch to tail of caudate nucleus
Post. communicating a.

Mammillary body

Oculomotor nerve branch

Posteromedial central a.

Posterior cerebral a. (postcommunical segment)

Superior cerebellar a.

Posterior cerebral a. (precommunical segment)

Basilar a.

Arteries of the brain

ARTERIES AT THE BASE OF SKULL (ARTERIAL CIRCLE OF WILLIS AND ITS BRANCHES, BASILAR ARTERY), INFERIOR (BRAIN) VIEW

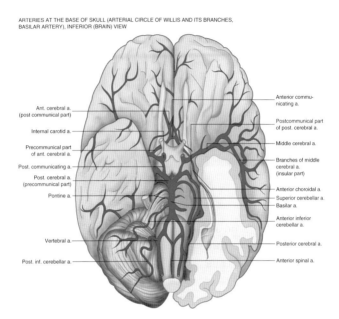

Ant. cerebral a. (post communical part)

Internal carotid a.

Precommunical part of ant. cerebral a.

Post. communicating a.

Post. cerebral a. (precommunical part)

Pontine a.

Vertebral a.

Post. inf. cerebellar a.

Anterior commu- nicating a.

Postcommunical part of post. cerebral a.

Middle cerebral a.

Branches of middle cerebral a. (insular part)

Anterior choroidal a.

Superior cerebellar a.

Basilar a.

Anterior inferior cerebellar a.

Posterior cerebral a.

Anterior spinal a.

Appendix 12
Stroke in the young and less common stroke diagnoses

Most strokes are caused by the mechanisms already described, i.e., cardioembolism, atherosclerosis, and small vessel disease, but at least 20% are due to other mechanisms. This is even more likely in younger patients (<40 years old), and older patients without atherosclerotic risk factors. The following is the approach to stroke diagnosis in younger patients and older patients in whom the cause remains obscure after the usual evaluation of the heart for sources of emboli and cerebral vessels for atherosclerosis, or who continue to have strokes despite standard treatment with antithrombotic agents and control of risk factors.

Tests to consider

- **Urine drug screen**.
- Go over home medications and supplements.
- **Hypercoagulable testing**. There is no consensus on when to do these, but certainly if there is a positive family history of clotting or previous history of DVT, pulmonary embolism, or miscarriage.

- Arterial thromboses:
  - antiphospholipid antibody panel (should include anti-cardiolipin IgM, anticardiolipin IgG)
  - lupus-anticoagulant (testing can be both mixing and Russell viper venom test)
  - hemoglobin electrophoresis
- Venous thromboses: same as above, plus:
  - protein C
  - protein S
  - antithrombin III
  - activated protein C (APC) resistance (biochemical test for Factor V Leiden, so you don't need the DNA test if you order this)
  - Factor V Leiden (DNA test)
  - Factor II (prothrombin gene) G20210A DNA test
- **Autoimmune laboratory testing**.
  - ESR, ANA, dsDNA, Complement 3, Complement 4, SS-A, SS-B (Sjögren's syndrome is associated with vasculitis)
- Fibrinogen level.
- Highly sensitive C-reactive protein (hs-CRP).

Note: Protein C, S, and antithrombin III can be falsely elevated acutely in stroke patients.

Causes

Extracranial causes

- arterial dissection (carotid, vertebral, aortic)
- aortic atheroma
- parodoxical embolus of venous clot through PFO
- air embolus (central venous catheter?)
- fibromuscular dysplasia

Intracranial causes

- cerebral venous thrombosis
- vasculitis (Primary CNS angiitis, polyarteritis nodosa, Takayasu's aortitis)
- infection
- moyamoya disease
- intravascular lymphoma

Hematological causes

- hypercoagulability
  - if no primary hematological problem is evident, look for underlying cancer
- collagen vascular disease
- drug abuse

Appendix 13
Brain death criteria

There are several hospital policies on the criteria for brain death, for example that published in 1968 by the Ad Hoc Committee of the Harvard Medical School to Examine the Definition of Brain Death.[109]

Nature of coma must be known

- Known structural disease or irreversible systemic metabolic cause that can explain the clinical picture.

Some causes must be ruled out

- Body temperature must be above 32.2 °C to rule out hypothermia.
- No chance of drug intoxication or neuromuscular blockade.
- Patient is not in shock.

Absence of cerebral and brain stem function

- Unresponsive to stimuli (i.e., no flexor or extensor posturing).
- Absent pupillary reflex.
- Absent caloric vestibular–ocular reflex.
- Absent corneal reflex.

- Absent gag reflex.
- Absent cough reflex.
- Areflexic: the limbs are flaccid, and there is no movement, although primitive withdrawal movements in response to local painful stimuli, mediated at a *spinal cord level,* can occur (i.e. not decorticate or decerebrate).
- Absent respiratory drive by apnea test.
- Some protocols require independent exams 6 hours apart by neurologist or neurosurgeon.
- Some protocols recommend 12-hour observation.

Apnea test

- Preoxygenate with 100% O_2. Get baseline arterial blood gas (pH and pCO_2 should be normal).
- Disconnect ventilator and give 100% O_2 by blow-by. Observe for spontaneous respirations. (If hypotension or arrhythmia occurs, immediately reconnect the ventilator.)
- After 10 minutes, or at earlier calculated interval, draw arterial blood gases, then reconnect the ventilator.
- Patient is apneic if $pCO_2 > 60$ mm Hg and there is no respiratory effort.

Confirmatory tests

These are not necessary to diagnose brain death. However, some protocols allow the diagnosis of brain death based on these studies. Therefore, they can be used in situations where it is not quite certain if the criteria are met on the physical exam, and also to bypass the prolonged observation period and need for repeated testing. They are frequently employed in patients who are candidates for organ donation.

- Cerebral blood flow studies with documentation of absent flow on one of the following:
  - angiogram;
  - nuclear medicine cerebral blood flow study.
- Electroencephalogram (EEG) with no physiologic brain activity.

Appendix 14
Neurological scales

Coma scale
- Glasgow coma scale

Hemorrhage scales
- ICH score
- Hunt and Hess scale for non-traumatic SAH
- World Federation of Neurological Surgeons (WFNS) scale for SAH

Long-term outcome scale
- Modified Rankin scale

Acute stroke scale
- National Institutes of Health stroke scale (NIHSS)

GLASGOW COMA SCALE

This scale is used in assessing depth of coma, and is therefore not useful for most stroke patients.

The scale adds three components: $(E + M + V) = 3 - 15$.

Response	Score	Characteristics
E: Eye opening		
None	1	Eyes always closed; not attributable to ocular swelling
To pain	2	Eyes open in response to painful stimulus
To speech	3	Eyes open in response to speech or shout
Spontaneous	4	Eyes open; does not imply intact awareness
M: Best motor response		
No response	1	No motor response to pain
Extension	2	Extension at elbow
Abnormal flexion	3	Includes preceding extension, stereotyped flexion posture, extreme wrist flexion, abduction of upper arm, flexion of fingers over thumb
Withdrawal	4	Normal flexor withdrawal; no localizing attempt to remove stimulus
Localizes pain	5	Attempt made to remove stimulus; e.g., hand moves above chin toward supraocular stimulus
Obeys commands	6	Follows simple commands

Response	Score	Characteristics
V: Best verbal response		
No response	1	No sounds
Incomprehensible	2	Moaning, groaning, grunting; incomprehensible
Inappropriate	3	Intelligible words, but not in a meaningful exchange; e.g., shouting, swearing
Confused	4	Responds to questions in conversational manner, but responses indicate varying degrees of disorientation and confusion
Oriented	5	Normal orientation to time, place, person

Source: G. Teasdale & B. Jennett, Assessment of coma and impaired consciousness: a practical scale. *Lancet* 1974; **2**: 81–4.[110] Copyright © 1974, with permission from Elsevier.

ICH SCORE

For prognosis in patients with ICH.

Component	ICH score points
GCS score	—
3–4	2
5–12	1
13–15	0
ICH volume, cm^3	—
≥30	1
<30	0
IVH	—
Yes	1
No	0
Infratentorial origin of ICH	—
Yes	1
No	0
Age, years	—
≥80	1
<80	0
Total ICH score (0–6)	—

Notes:

GCS score: Glasgow coma score on initial presentation (or after resuscitation)

ICH volume: volume on initial CT calculated using ABC/2 method (see Appendix 1)

IVH: presence of any intraventricular hemorrhage on initial CT

Source: J. C. Hemphill, D. C. Bonovich, L. Besmertis, G. T. Manley, & S. C. Johnston, The ICH score: a simple, reliable grading scale for intracerebral hemorrhage. *Stroke* 2001; **32**: 891–7.[84] Reproduced with permission from Lippincott Williams & Wilkins.

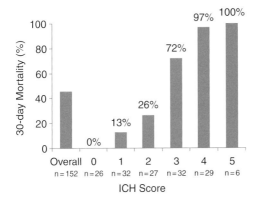

Outcome based on ICH score

Source: J. C. Hemphill, D. C. Bonovich, L. Besmertis, G. T. Manley, & S. C. Johnston, The ICH score: a simple, reliable grading scale for intracerebral hemorrhage. *Stroke* 2001; **32**: 891–7.[84] Reproduced with permission from Lippincott Williams & Wilkins.

HUNT AND HESS SCALE FOR NON-TRAUMATIC SAH

This scale is used for assessing the severity and prognosis of patients with SAH.

Grade	
1	Asymptomatic, mild headache, slight nuchal rigidity
2	Moderate to severe headache, nuchal rigidity
	No neurologic deficit other than CN palsy
3	Drowsiness/confusion
	Mild focal neurologic deficit
4	Stupor
	Moderate – severe hemiparesis
5	Coma
	Decerebrate posturing

Source: W. E. Hunt & R. M. Hess, Surgical risk as related to time of intervention in the repair of intracranial aneurysms. *J. Neurosurg.* 1968; **28**: 14–20.[111] Reproduced with permission from the *Journal of Neurosurgery.*

WFNS SCALE FOR SAH

Another scale used in prognosis for SAH. WFNS = World Federation of Neurological Surgeons.

Grade	
1	GCS 15 = good grade
2	GCS 14–13, with no motor deficit = fair grade
3	GCS 14–13, with hemiparesis or aphasia = tending to poor grade
4	GCS 12–8, with or without hemiparesis or aphasia = poor grade
5	GCS < 8, with or without hemiparesis or aphasia = moribund patient

Source: G. M. Teasdale, C. G. Drake, W. Hunt, *et al.*, A universal subarachnoid hemorrhage scale: report of a committee of the World Federation of Neurosurgical Societies. *J. Neurol. Neurosurg. Psychiatry* 1988; **51**: 1457.[112] Reproduced with permission from BMJ Publishing Group.

MODIFIED RANKIN SCALE

A scale commonly used to measure disability or dependence in activities of daily living.[113–115]

Score	Description
0	No symptoms at all
1	No significant disability despite symptoms; able to carry out all usual duties and activities
2	Slight disability; unable to carry out all previous activities, but able to look after own affairs without assistance
3	Moderate disability; requiring some help, but able to walk without assistance
4	Moderately severe disability; unable to walk without assistance and unable to attend to own bodily needs without assistance
5	Severe disability; bedridden, incontinent and requiring constant nursing care and attention
6	Dead
Total	(0–6): ___

NATIONAL INSTITUTES OF HEALTH STROKE SCALE (NIHSS)

This is the most commonly used scale for assessing the severity of stroke.[116,117] It is most useful for the initial grading of stroke severity and for following its course, and less useful for determining outcome since it does not measure function. It has been proven reliable and reproducible, **but requires training and certification**.

The training can be obtained through the American Stroke Association's website (www.strokeassociation.org) as well as other sites.

The NIHSS forms are available at the NIH website:

- www.ninds.nih.gov/doctors/NIH_Stroke_Scale.pdf
- www.ninds.nih.gov/doctors/NIH_Stroke_Scale_Booklet.pdf

Guides to scoring to improve consistency:

- Score the first response that the patient makes.
- Score only if abnormality is present for some items (e.g., ataxia is absent if the patient is hemiplegic).
- Record what the patient does, not what you think the patient can do.

The pictures at the end are used for standardizing the aphasia exam. Have the patient name the objects and describe what is happening in the picture.

1a. Level of consciousness	0 = **Alert**: keenly responsive. **1a:**
A 3 is scored only if the patient makes no movement (other than reflexive posturing) in response to noxious stimulation.	1 = **Not alert, but arousable** by minor stimulation to obey, answer, or respond.
	2 = **Not alert, obtunded**. Requires repeated stimulation to attend, or requires strong or painful stimulation to make movements.
	3 = **Coma**. Responds only with reflex motor or autonomic effects, or totally unresponsive.
1b. LOC questions **Ask the month and his/her age.**	0 = **Answers both questions correctly.** **1b:**
Aphasic and stuporous patients who do not comprehend the questions → score 2.	1 = **Answers one question correctly.**
Endotracheal intubation, severe dysarthria, language barrier and problems other than aphasia → score 1. Grade the initial answer.	2 = **Answers neither question correctly.**
1c. LOC commands **Open and close the eyes.**	0 = **Performs both tasks correctly.** **1c:**
Open and close the non-paretic hand.	1 = **Performs one task correctly.**
Only the first attempt is scored.	2 = **Performs neither task correctly.**

2. Best gaze

Only voluntary or reflexive (oculocephalic) eye movements are tested. Caloric testing is not done.

A conjugate deviation of the eyes that can be overcome by voluntary or reflexive activity → score 1.

Isolated cranial nerve paresis (CN III, IV or VI) → score 1. Gaze is testable in all aphasic patients.

0 = **Normal**.

1 = **Partial gaze palsy**. Gaze is abnormal in one or both eyes, but forced deviation or total gaze paresis are not present.

2 = **Forced deviation**, or total gaze paresis not overcome by the oculocephalic maneuver.

2: —

3. Visual fields

Both upper and lower quadrants are tested by confrontation, using finger counting.

Unable to make proper response (e.g., aphasia, obtundation) → use blink to visual threat from the side.

Unilateral blindness or enucleation → test in the remaining eye.

0 = **No visual loss**.

1 = **Partial hemianopia** (e.g., quadrantanopia, extinction to bilateral simultaneous stimulation).

2 = **Complete hemianopia**.

3 = **Bilateral hemianopia** (blind, including cortical blindness).

3: —

4. Facial palsy

Ask, or use pantomime to encourage the patient to show teeth or raise eyebrows and close eyes.

Poorly responsive or noncomprehending patient → use symmetry of grimace in response to noxious stimuli.

0 = **Normal** symmetrical movement.

1 = **Minor paralysis** (flattened nasolabial fold, asymmetry on smiling).

2 = **Partial paralysis** (total or near total paralysis of lower face).

4: —

	3 = Complete paralysis of one or both sides (absence of facial movement in the upper and lower face).	
5 & 6. Motor arm and leg	**0 = No drift.** Limb holds 90 (or 45) degrees for full 10 seconds (arm) or 30 degrees for 5 seconds (leg).	**5a. Left arm:**
The limb is placed in the appropriate position: **Arm** extended with palms down 90 degrees (if sitting) or 45 degrees (if supine) for 10 seconds.		**5b. Right arm:**
Leg extended at 30 degrees (always tested supine) for 5 seconds.	**1 = Drift.** Limb drifts down before full 10 seconds (arm) or 5 seconds (leg); does not hit bed or other support.	**6a. Left leg:**
The aphasic patient is encouraged using urgency in the voice and pantomime but not noxious stimulation.	**2 = Some effort against gravity.** Limb cannot get to or maintain position and drifts down to bed, but has some effort against gravity.	**6b. Right leg:**
	3 = No effort against gravity. Limb falls.	
	4 = No movement.	
	9 = Amputation or joint fusion. Do not add to total score. Explain.	
7. Limb ataxia	**0 = Absent.**	**7:**
The **finger–nose–finger** and **heel–shin** tests are performed on both sides, and ataxia is scored *only if present out of proportion to weakness.*	**1 = Present in one limb.**	
	2 = Present in two limbs.	

In case of visual defect, insure testing is done in intact visual field.

Ataxia is absent in the patient who cannot understand or is paralyzed.

In case of blindness test by touching nose from extended arm position.

9 = Amputation or joint fusion. Do not add to total score. Explain.

8. Sensory

Sensation or grimace to pinprick, or withdrawal from noxious stimulus in the obtunded or aphasic patient. Only sensory loss attributed to stroke is scored as abnormal. Test as many body areas (arms [not hands], legs, trunk, face) as needed to be accurate.

Score 2 only when a severe or total loss of sensation can be clearly demonstrated.

Brainstem stroke with bilateral loss of sensation → score 2. Patient does not respond and is quadriplegic → score 2. Coma (item 1a = 3) → score 2.

8: ____

0 = **Normal**. No sensory loss.

1 = **Mild to moderate sensory loss**. Patient feels pinprick is less sharp or is dull on the affected side; or there is a loss of superficial pain with pinprick but patient is aware he/she is being touched.

2 = **Severe to total sensory loss**. Patient is not aware of being touched in the face, arm, or leg.

9. Best language

The patient is asked to describe what is happening in the picture, to name the items on the naming sheet, and to read from the list of sentences. Comprehension is judged

9: ____

0 = **No aphasia, normal**.

1 = **Mild to moderate aphasia**. Some obvious loss of fluency or facility of comprehension, without significant

from responses here as well as to all of the commands in the preceding general neurological exam.

Visual loss interferes with the tests → ask patient to identify objects placed in the hand, repeat, and produce speech.

Intubated patient → ask patient to write responses.

Coma (item 1a = 3) → score 3.

Give adequate time, but only the first response is measured.

limitation on ideas expressed or form of expression.

2 = **Severe aphasia**. All communication is through fragmentary expression; great need for inference, questioning, and guessing by the listener.

3 = **Mute, global aphasia**. No usable speech or auditory comprehension.

10. Dysarthria

A sample of speech must be obtained by asking the patient to read or repeat words from the list. If the patient has severe aphasia, the clarity of articulation of spontaneous speech can be rated.

Mute due to aphasis → score 2.

Intubation or physical barrier → do not score.

10: ⎯

0 = **Normal**.

1 = **Mild to moderate**. Patient slurs at least some words and, at worst, can be understood with some difficulty.

2 = **Severe**. Patient's speech is so slurred as to be unintelligible in the absence of or out of proportion to any dysphasia, or is mute/anarthric.

9 = Intubated or other physical barrier. Do not add to total score. Explain.

11. Extinction and inattention

Sufficient information to identify neglect may be obtained during the prior testing.

Aphasia but appears to attend to both sides → normal.

Since the abnormality is scored only if present, the item is never untestable.

0 = No abnormality.

1 = Present. Visual, tactile, auditory, spatial, or personal inattention or extinction to bilateral simultaneous stimulation in one of the sensory modalities.

2 = Profound hemi-inattention or hemi-inattention to more than one modality. Does not recognize own hand or orients to only one side of space.

11:

—

For the dysarthria exam, have the patient say the following words

MAMA

TIP-TOP

FIFTY-FIFTY

THANKS

HUCKLEBERRY

BASEBALL PLAYER

CATERPILLAR

For the aphasia exam, have the patient name
the objects pictured below

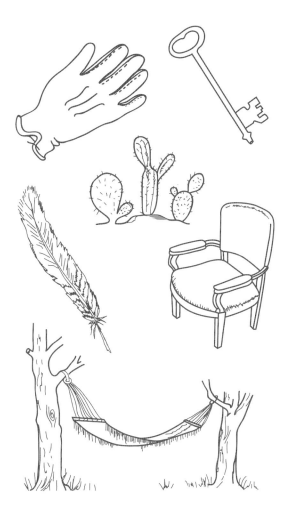

For the aphasia exam, have the patient read the following sentences

You know how.

Down to earth.

I got home from work.

Near the table in the dining room.

They heard him speak on the radio last night.

For the aphasia exam, have the patient describe
what is happening in the following picture

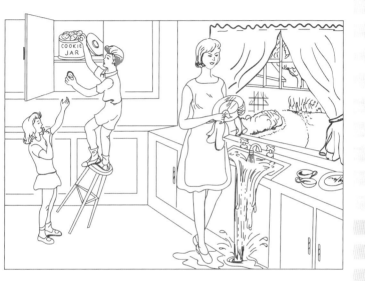

Recommended reading

Textbooks

Mohr, J. P., Choi, D., Grotta, J. C., Weir, B., & Wolf, P. *Stroke: Pathophysiology, Diagnosis, & Management.* 4th edn. Philadelphia, PA: Churchill Livingstone, 2004.

Warlow, C. P., Dennis, M. S., van Gijn, J., & Hankey, G. J. *Stroke.* 2nd edn. Oxford: Blackwell, 2001.

Caplan, L. R. *Caplan's Stroke: a Clinical Approach.* 3rd edn. Boston, MA: Butterworth-Heinemann, 2000.

Adams, H. P., Jr., Hachinski, V. & Norris, J. W. *Ischemic Cerebrovascular Disease.* Contemporary Neurology Series. Oxford: Oxford University Press, 2001.

Bogousslavsky, J. and Caplan, L. *Stroke Syndromes.* 2nd edn. Cambridge: Cambridge University Press, 2001.

Bogousslavsky, J. and Caplan, L. *Uncommon Causes of Stroke.* 2nd edn. Cambridge: Cambridge University Press, 2001.

Guidelines

AHA/ASA scientific statement. Guidelines for the early management of patients with ischemic stroke. *Stroke* 2005; **36**: 916–23.

ASA scientific statement. Guidelines for the management of spontaneous intracerebral hemorrhage. *Stroke* 1999; **30**: 905–15.

AHA scientific statement. Guidelines for the management of aneurysmal subarachnoid hemorrhage. *Circulation* 1994; **90**: 2592–605.

AHA scientific statement. Recommendations for the management of patients with unruptured intracranial aneurysms. *Circulation* 2000; **102**: 2300–8.

European Stroke Initiative recommendations for stroke management: update 2003. *Cerebrovasc. Dis.* 2003; **16**: 311–37.

European Stroke Initiative. Recommendations for stroke management. http://www.eusi-stroke.com/recommendations/rc_overview.shtml.

Bates, B., Choi, J. Y., Duncan, P. W., *et al.* Veterans Affairs/Department of Defense clinical practice guideline for the management of adult stroke rehabilitation care: executive summary [AHA/ASA-endorsed practice guidelines]. *Stroke* 2005; **36**: 2049–56.

Sacco, R. L., Adams, R., Albers, G., *et al.* Guidelines for prevention of stroke in patients with ischemic stroke or transient ischemic attack. *Stroke* 2006; **37**: 577–617.

Stroke prevention

Albers, G. W., Amarenco, P., Easton, J. D., Sacco, R. L., & Teal, P. Antithrombotics. *Chest* 2001; **119**: 300S–320S

Gorelick, P. B. Stroke prevention therapy beyond antithrombotics: unifying mechanisms in ischemic stroke pathogenesis and implications for therapy. *Stroke* 2002; **33**: 862–75.

Thrombolysis

Tissue plasminogen activator for acute ischemic stroke. The National Institute of Neurological Disorders and Stroke rt-PA Stroke Study Group. *N. Engl. J. Med.* 1995; **333**: 1581–8.

Lyden, P. D. *Thrombolytic Therapy for Acute Stroke.* 2nd edn. Totowa, NJ: Humana Press, 2005.

ICH

Qureshi, A. I., Tuhrim, S., Broderick, J. P., Batjer, H. H., Hondo, H., & Hanley, D. F. Spontaneous intracerebral hemorrhage. *N. Engl. J. Med.* 2001; **344**: 1450–60.

Atrial fibrillation

Hart, R. G., Halperin, J. L., Pearce, L. A., *et al.* Lessons from the Stroke Prevention in Atrial Fibrillation trials. *Ann. Intern. Med.* 2003; **138**: 831–8.

Radiology

Parizel, P. M., Makkat, S., Van Miert, E., Van Goethem, J. W., van den Hauwe, L., & De Schepper, A. M. Intracranial hemorrhage: principles of CT and MRI interpretation. *Eur. Radiol.* 2001; **11**: 1770–83.

AVM

Fleetwood, I. G. & Steinberg, G. K. Arteriovenous malformations. *Lancet* 2002; **359**: 863–73.

SAH/Aneurysm

Van Gijn, J. & Rinkel, G. J. E. Subarachnoid haemorrhage: diagnosis, causes and managment. *Brain* 2001; **124**: 249–78.

References

1. Adams, H. P., Jr., Adams, R. J., Brott, T., *et al.* Guidelines for the early management of patients with ischemic stroke: a scientific statement from the Stroke Council of the American Stroke Association. *Stroke* 2003; **34**: 1056–83.

2. Adams, H., Adams, R., Del Zoppo, G., & Goldstein, L. B. Guidelines for the early management of patients with ischemic stroke: 2005 guidelines update. A Scientific Statement from the Stroke Council of the American Heart Association/American Stroke Association. *Stroke* 2005; **36**: 916–23.

3. The International Stroke Trial (IST): a randomised trial of aspirin, subcutaneous heparin, both, or neither among 19435 patients with acute ischaemic stroke. International Stroke Trial Collaborative Group. *Lancet* 1997; **349**: 1569–81.

4. CAST: randomised placebo-controlled trial of early aspirin use in 20,000 patients with acute ischaemic stroke. CAST (Chinese Acute Stroke Trial) Collaborative Group. *Lancet* 1997; **349**: 1641–9.

5. Berge, E., Abdelnoor, M., Nakstad, P. H., & Sandset, P. M. Low molecular-weight heparin versus aspirin in patients with acute ischaemic stroke and atrial fibrillation: a double-blind randomised study. HAEST Study Group. Heparin in Acute Embolic Stroke Trial. *Lancet* 2000; **355**: 1205–10.

6. Hart, R. G., Palacio, S., & Pearce, L. A. Atrial fibrillation, stroke, and acute antithrombotic therapy: analysis of randomized clinical trials. *Stroke* 2002; **33**: 2722–7.

7. Albers, G. W., Amarenco, P., Easton, J. D., Sacco, R. L., & Teal, P. Antithrombotic and thrombolytic therapy for ischemic stroke: the Seventh ACCP Conference on Antithrombotic and Thrombolytic

Therapy. *Chest* 2004; **126** (3 suppl.): 483S–512S. http://www.chestjournal.org/cgi/reprint/126/3_suppl/483S.

8. Adams, H. P., Jr., Bendixen, B. H., Kappelle, L. J., *et al.* Classification of subtype of acute ischemic stroke. Definitions for use in a multicenter clinical trial. TOAST. Trial of Org 10172 in Acute Stroke Treatment. *Stroke* 1993; **24**: 35–41.

9. U-King-Im, J. M., Trivedi, R. A., Graves, M. J., *et al.* Contrast-enhanced MR angiography for carotid disease: diagnostic and potential clinical impact. *Neurology* 2004; **62**: 1282–90.

10. Petty, G. W., Brown, R. D., Jr., Whisnant, J. P., Sicks, J. D., O'Fallon, W. M., & Wiebers, D. O. Survival and recurrence after first cerebral infarction: a population-based study in Rochester, Minnesota, 1975 through 1989. *Neurology* 1998; **50**: 208–16.

11. Hartmann, A., Rundek, T., Mast, H., *et al.* Mortality and causes of death after first ischemic stroke: the Northern Manhattan Stroke Study. *Neurology* 2001; **57**: 2000–5.

12. Bravata, D. M., Ho, S. Y., Brass, L. M., Concato, J., Scinto, J., & Meehan, T. P. Long-term mortality in cerebrovascular disease. *Stroke* 2003; **34**: 699–704.

13. Dewey, H. M., Sturm, J., Donnan, G. A., Macdonell, R. A., McNeil, J. J., & Thrift, A. G. Incidence and outcome of subtypes of ischaemic stroke: initial results from the North East Melbourne stroke incidence study (NEMESIS). *Cerebrovasc. Dis.* 2003; **15**: 133–9.

14. The National Institute of Neurological Disorders and Stroke rt-PA Stroke Study Group. Tissue plasminogen activator for acute ischemic stroke. *N. Engl. J. Med.* 1995; **333**: 1581–7.

15. Marler, J. R., Tilley, B. C., Lu, M., *et al.* Early stroke treatment associated with better outcome: the NINDS rt-PA stroke study. *Neurology* 2000; **55**: 1649–55.

16. Generalized efficacy of t-PA for acute stroke. Subgroup analysis of the NINDS t-PA Stroke Trial. *Stroke* 1997; **28**: 2119–25.

17. Patel, S. C., Levine, S. R., Tilley, B. C., *et al.* Lack of clinical significance of early ischemic changes on computed tomography in acute stroke. *JAMA* 2001; **286**: 2830–8.

18. Combined intravenous and intra-arterial recanalization for acute ischemic stroke: the Interventional Management of Stroke Study. *Stroke* 2004; **35**: 904–11.

19. Hacke, W., Donnan, G., Fieschi, C., *et al.* Association of outcome with early stroke treatment: pooled analysis of ATLANTIS, ECASS, and NINDS rt-PA stroke trials. *Lancet* 2004; **363**: 768–74.

20. Smith, W. C., Sung, G., Starkman, S., *et al.* Safety and efficacy of mechanical embolectomy in acute ischemic stroke: results of the MERCI trial. *Stroke* 2005; **36**: 1432–8.

21. Saxena, R., Lewis, S., Berge, E., Sandercock, P. A., & Koudstaal, P. J. Risk of early death and recurrent stroke and effect of heparin in 3169 patients with acute ischemic stroke and atrial fibrillation in the International Stroke Trial. *Stroke* 2001; **32**: 2333–7.

22. Kang, D. W., Latour, L. L., Chalela, J. A., Dambrosia, J., & Warach, S. Early ischemic lesion recurrence within a week after acute ischemic stroke. *Ann. Neurol.* 2003; **54**: 66–74.

23. Lovett, J. K., Coull, A. J., & Rothwell, P. M. Early risk of recurrence by subtype of ischemic stroke in population-based incidence studies. *Neurology* 2004; **62**: 569–73.

24. Fiorelli, M., Bastianello, S., von Kummer, R., *et al.* Hemorrhagic transformation within 36 hours of a cerebral infarct: relationships with early clinical deterioration and 3-month outcome in the European Cooperative Acute Stroke Study I (ECASS I) cohort. *Stroke* 1999; **30**: 2280–4.

25. Lees, K. R., Zivin, J. A., Ashwood, T., *et al.* for the Stroke–Acute Ischemic NXY Treatment (SAINT I) Trial Investigators. NXY-059 for acute ischemic stroke. *N. Engl. J. Med.* 2006; **354**: 588–600.

26. Schneider, L. S., Dagerman, K. S., & Insel, P. Risk of death with atypical antipsychotic drug treatment for dementia: meta-analysis of randomized placebo-controlled trials. *JAMA* 2005; **294**: 1934–43.

27. Sacco, R. L., Adams, R., Albers, G., *et al.* Guidelines for prevention of stroke in patients with ischemic stroke or transient ischemic attack. *Stroke* 2006; **37**: 577–617.

28. SHEP Cooperative Research Group. Prevention of stroke by antihypertensive drug treatment in older persons with isolated systolic hypertension. Final results of the Systolic Hypertension in the Elderly Program (SHEP). *JAMA* 1991; **265**: 3255–64.

29. Yusuf, S., Sleight, P., Pogue, J., Bosch, J., Davies, R., & Dagenais, G. Effects of an angiotensin-converting-enzyme inhibitor, ramipril, on cardiovascular events in high-risk patients. The Heart Outcomes

Prevention Evaluation Study Investigators. *N. Engl. J. Med.* 2000; **342**: 145–53.

30. Randomised trial of a perindopril based blood-pressure-lowering regimen among 6,105 individuals with previous stroke or transient ischaemic attack. *Lancet* 2001; **358**: 1033–41.

31. Major outcomes in high-risk hypertensive patients randomized to angiotensin-converting enzyme inhibitor or calcium channel blocker vs diuretic: The Antihypertensive and Lipid-Lowering Treatment to Prevent Heart Attack Trial (ALLHAT). *JAMA* 2002; **288**: 2981–97.

32. MRC/BHF Heart Protection Study of cholesterol lowering with simvastatin in 20,536 high-risk individuals: a randomised placebo-controlled trial. *Lancet* 2002; **360**: 7–22.

33. Grundy, S. M., Cleeman, J. I., Merz, C. N., *et al.* Implications of recent clinical trials for the National Cholesterol Education Program Adult Treatment Panel III guidelines. *Circulation* 2004; **110**: 227–39.

34. Toole, J. F., Malinow, M. R., Chambless, L. E., *et al.* Lowering homocysteine in patients with ischemic stroke to prevent recurrent stroke, myocardial infarction, and death: the Vitamin Intervention for Stroke Prevention (VISP) randomized controlled trial. *JAMA* 2004; **291**: 565–75.

35. Viscoli, C. M., Brass, L. M., Kernan, W. N., Sarrel, P. M., Suissa, S., & Horwitz, R. I. A clinical trial of estrogen-replacement therapy after ischemic stroke. *N. Engl. J. Med.* 2001; **345**: 1243–9.

36. Anderson, G. L., Limacher, M., Assaf, A. R., *et al.* Effects of conjugated equine estrogen in postmenopausal women with hysterectomy: the Women's Health Initiative randomized controlled trial. *JAMA* 2004; **291**: 1701–12.

37. Rossouw, J. E., Anderson, G. L., Prentice, R. L., *et al.* Risks and benefits of estrogen plus progestin in healthy postmenopausal women: principal results from the Women's Health Initiative randomized controlled trial. *JAMA* 2002; **288**: 321–33.

38. Antiplatelet Trialists' Collaboration. Collaborative overview of randomised trials of antiplatelet therapy. I: Prevention of death, myocardial infarction, and stroke by prolonged antiplatelet therapy in various categories of patients. *BMJ* 1994; **308**: 81–106.

39. Diener, H. C., Cunha, L., Forbes, C., Sivenius, J., Smets, P., & Lowenthal, A. European Stroke Prevention Study. 2. Dipyridamole and

acetylsalicylic acid in the secondary prevention of stroke. *J. Neurol. Sci.* 1996; **143**: 1–13.

40. The ESPS Group. The European Stroke Prevention Study (ESPS): principal end-points. *Lancet* 1987; **2**: 1351–4.

41. CAPRIE Steering Committee. A randomised, blinded, trial of clopidogrel versus aspirin in patients at risk of ischaemic events (CAPRIE). *Lancet* 1996; **348**: 1329–39.

42. Diener, H. C., Bogousslavsky, J., Brass, L. M., *et al.* Aspirin and clopidogrel compared with clopidogrel alone after recent ischaemic stroke or transient ischaemic attack in high-risk patients (MATCH): randomised, double-blind, placebo-controlled trial. *Lancet* 2004; **364**: 331–7.

43. Bhatt, D. L., Fox, K. A. A., Hacke, W., *et al.* Clopidogrel and aspirin versus aspirin alone for the prevention of atherothrombotic events. *N. Engl. J. Med.* 2006; **354**: 1706–17.

44. Hart, R. G., Halperin, J. L., Pearce, L. A., *et al.* Lessons from the Stroke Prevention in Atrial Fibrillation trials. *Ann. Intern. Med.* 2003; **138**: 831–8.

45. Saxena, R. & Koudstaal, P. Anticoagulants versus antiplatelet therapy for preventing stroke in patients with nonrheumatic atrial fibrillation and a history of stroke or transient ischemic attack. *Cochrane Database Syst. Rev.* 2004(4): CD000187.

46. Ferro, J. M. Cardioembolic stroke: an update. *Lancet Neurol.* 2003; **2**: 177–88.

47. Amarenco, P., Cohen, A., Tzourio, C., *et al.* Atherosclerotic disease of the aortic arch and the risk of ischemic stroke. *N. Engl. J. Med.* 1994; **331**: 1474–9.

48. Blackshear, J. L., Zabalgoitia, M., Pennock, G., *et al.* Warfarin safety and efficacy in patients with thoracic aortic plaque and atrial fibrillation. SPAF TEE Investigators. Stroke Prevention and Atrial Fibrillation. Transesophageal echocardiography. *Am. J. Cardiol.* 1999; **83**: 453–5, A9.

49. Mohr, J. P. Anticoagulation for stroke prevention: yes, no, maybe. *Cleve. Clin. J. Med.* 2004; **71** (Suppl. 1): S52–6.

50. Homma, S., Sacco, R. L., Di Tullio, M. R., Sciacca, R. R., & Mohr, J. P. Effect of medical treatment in stroke patients with patent foramen ovale: patent foramen ovale in Cryptogenic Stroke Study. *Circulation* 2002; **105**: 2625–31.

51. Chimowitz, M. I., Lynn, M. J., Howlett-Smith, H., *et al.* Comparison of warfarin and aspirin for symptomatic intracranial arterial stenosis. *N. Engl. J. Med.* 2005; **352**: 1305–16.

52. Mohr, J. P., Thompson, J. L., Lazar, R. M., *et al.* A comparison of warfarin and aspirin for the prevention of recurrent ischemic stroke. *N. Engl. J. Med.* 2001; **345**: 1444–51.

53. Levine, S. R., Brey, R. L., Tilley, B. C., *et al.* Antiphospholipid antibodies and subsequent thrombo-occlusive events in patients with ischemic stroke. *JAMA* 2004; **291**: 576–84.

54. Chobanian, A. V., Bakris, G. L., Black, H. R., *et al.* The Seventh Report of the Joint National Committee on Prevention, Detection, Evaluation, and Treatment of High Blood Pressure: the JNC 7 report. *JAMA* 2003; **289**: 2560–72.

55. Dahlof, B., Devereux, R. B., Kjeldsen, S. E., *et al.* Cardiovascular morbidity and mortality in the Losartan Intervention For Endpoint reduction in hypertension study (LIFE): a randomised trial against atenolol. *Lancet* 2002; **359**: 995–1003.

56. Psaty, B. M., Lumley, T., Furberg, C. D., *et al.* Health outcomes associated with various antihypertensive therapies used as first-line agents: a network meta-analysis. *JAMA* 2003; **289**: 2534–44.

57. Barnett, H. J. Decision-making for carotid endarterectomy: the trials are only the start. *Can. J. Neurol. Sci.* 2002; **29**: 302–4.

58. Barnett, H. J., Taylor, D. W., Eliasziw, M., *et al.* Benefit of carotid endarterectomy in patients with symptomatic moderate or severe stenosis. North American Symptomatic Carotid Endarterectomy Trial Collaborators. *N. Engl. J. Med.* 1998; **339**: 1415–25.

59. Executive Committee for the Asymptomatic Carotid Atherosclerosis Study. Endarterectomy for asymptomatic carotid artery stenosis. *JAMA* 1995; **273**: 1421–8.

60. Halliday, A., Mansfield, A., Marro, J., *et al.* Prevention of disabling and fatal strokes by successful carotid endarterectomy in patients without recent neurological symptoms: randomised controlled trial. *Lancet* 2004; **363**: 1491–502.

61. Yadav, J. S., Wholey, M. H., Kuntz, R. E., *et al.* Protected carotid-artery stenting versus endarterectomy in high-risk patients. *N. Engl. J. Med.* 2004; **351**: 1493–501.

62. Rothwell, P. M., Eliasziw, M., Gutnikov, S. A., Warlow, C. P., & Barnett, H. J. Endarterectomy for symptomatic carotid stenosis in relation to clinical subgroups and timing of surgery. *Lancet* 2004; **363**: 915–24.

63. Rothwell, P. M., Eliasziw, M., Gutnikov, S. A., Warlow, C. P., & Barnett, H. J. Sex difference in the effect of time from symptoms to surgery on benefit from carotid endarterectomy for transient ischemic attack and nondisabling stroke. *Stroke* 2004; **35**: 2855–61.

64. Bond, R., Rerkasem, K., & Rothwell, P. M. Systematic review of the risks of carotid endarterectomy in relation to the clinical indication for and timing of surgery. *Stroke* 2003; **34**: 2290–301.

65. Grubb, R. L., Jr., Powers, W. J., Derdeyn, C. P., Adams, H. P., Jr., & Clarke, W. R. The carotid occlusion surgery study. *Neurosurg. Focus* 2003; **14** (3): e9.

66. Grubb, R. L., Jr., Derdeyn, C. P., Fritsch, S. M., *et al.* Importance of hemodynamic factors in the prognosis of symptomatic carotid occlusion. *JAMA* 1998; **280**: 1055–60.

67. Vernieri, F., Pasqualetti, P., Passarelli, F., Rossini, P. M., & Silvestrini, M. Outcome of carotid artery occlusion is predicted by cerebrovascular reactivity. *Stroke* 1999; **30**: 593–8.

68. Yonemura, K., Kimura, K., Minematsu, K., Uchino, M., & Yamaguchi, T. Small centrum ovale infarcts on diffusion-weighted magnetic resonance imaging. *Stroke* 2002; **33**: 1541–4.

69. Landau, W. M. Clinical neuromythology VI. Au clair de lacune: holy, wholly, holey logic. *Neurology* 1989; **39**: 725–30.

70. Perry, H. M., Jr., Davis, B. R., Price, T. R., *et al.* Effect of treating isolated systolic hypertension on the risk of developing various types and subtypes of stroke: the Systolic Hypertension in the Elderly Program (SHEP). *JAMA* 2000; **284**: 465–71.

71. Chen, C. J., Tseng, Y. C., Lee, T. H., Hsu, H. L., & See, L. C. Multisection CT angiography compared with catheter angiography in diagnosing vertebral artery dissection. *AJNR Am. J. Neuroradiol.* 2004; **25**: 769–74.

72. Touze, E., Gauvrit, J. Y., Moulin, T., Meder, J. F., Bracard, S., & Mas, J. L. Risk of stroke and recurrent dissection after a cervical artery dissection: a multicenter study. *Neurology* 2003; **61**: 1347–51.

73. Overell, J. R., Bone, I., & Lees, K. R. Interatrial septal abnormalities and stroke: a meta-analysis of case–control studies. *Neurology* 2000; **55**: 1172–9.

74. Messe, S. R., Silverman, I. E., Kizer, J. R., *et al.* Practice parameter: recurrent stroke with patent foramen ovale and atrial septal aneurysm. Report of the Quality Standards Subcommittee of the American Academy of Neurology. *Neurology* 2004; **62**: 1042–50.

75. Albers, G. W., Caplan, L. R., Easton, J. D., *et al*. Transient ischemic attack: proposal for a new definition. *N. Engl. J. Med.* 2002; **347**: 1713–16.

76. Johnston, S. C., Gress, D. R., Browner, W. S., & Sidney, S. Short-term prognosis after emergency department diagnosis of TIA. *JAMA* 2000; **284**: 2901–6.

77. Johnston, S. C. & Sidney, S. Validation of a 4-point prediction rule to stratify short-term stroke risk after TIA [abstract]. *Stroke* 2005; **36**: 430. [Presentation, International Stroke Meeting, February 2006.]

78. Qureshi, A. I., Tuhrim, S., Broderick, J. P., Batjer, H. H., Hondo, H., & Hanley, D. F. Spontaneous intracerebral hemorrhage. *N. Engl. J. Med.* 2001; **344**: 1450–60.

79. Mendelow, A. D., Gregson, B. A., Fernandes, H. M., *et al*. Early surgery versus initial conservative treatment in patients with spontaneous supratentorial intracerebral haematomas in the International Surgical Trial in Intracerebral Haemorrhage (STICH): a randomised trial. *Lancet* 2005; **365**: 387–97.

80. Broderick, J. P., Adams, H. P., Jr., Barsan, W., *et al*. Guidelines for the management of spontaneous intracerebral hemorrhage: a statement for healthcare professionals from a special writing group of the Stroke Council, American Heart Association. *Stroke* 1999; **30**: 905–15.

81. Brott, T., Broderick, J., Kothari, R., *et al*. Early hemorrhage growth in patients with intracerebral hemorrhage. *Stroke* 1997; **28**: 1–5.

82. Mayer, S. A., Brun, N. C., Begtrup, K., *et al*. Recombinant activated factor VII for acute intracerebral hemorrhage. *N. Engl. J. Med.* 2005; **352**: 777–85.

83. Broderick, J. P., Brott, T. G., Duldner, J. E., Tomsick, T., & Huster, G. Volume of intracerebral hemorrhage: a powerful and easy-to-use predictor of 30-day mortality. *Stroke* 1993; **24**: 987–93.

84. Hemphill, J. C., Bonovich, D. C., Besmertis, L., Manley, G. T., & Johnston, S. C. The ICH score: a simple, reliable grading scale for intracerebral hemorrhage. *Stroke* 2001; **32**: 891–7.

85. Mayberg, M. R., Batjer, H. H., Dacey, R. *et al*. Guidelines for the management of aneurysmal subarachnoid hemorrhage. A statement for healthcare professionals from a special writing group of the Stroke Council, American Heart Association. *Stroke* 1994; **25**: 2315–28.

86. Molyneux, A., Kerr, R., Stratton, I., *et al*. International Subarachnoid Aneurysm Trial (ISAT) of neurosurgical clipping versus endovascular

coiling in 2143 patients with ruptured intracranial aneurysms: a randomised trial. *Lancet* 2002; **360**: 1267–74.

87. van den Bergh, W. M., Algra, A., van Kooten, F., *et al.* Magnesium sulfate in aneurysmal subarachnoid hemorrhage: a randomized controlled trial. *Stroke* 2005; **36**: 1011–15.

88. Longstreth, W. T., Jr., Nelson, L. M., Koepsell, T. D., & van Belle, G. Clinical course of spontaneous subarachnoid hemorrhage: a population-based study in King County, Washington. *Neurology* 1993; **43**: 712–18.

89. Kassell, N. F., Torner, J. C., Jane, J. A., Haley, E. C., Jr., & Adams, H. P. The International Cooperative Study on the Timing of Aneurysm Surgery. Part 2: surgical results. *J. Neurosurg.* 1990; **73**: 37–47.

90. International Study of Unruptured Intracranial Aneurysms Investigators. Unruptured intracranial aneurysms: risk of rupture and risks of surgical intervention. *N. Engl. J. Med.* 1998; **339**: 1725–33.

91. Wiebers, D. O., Whisnant, J. P., Huston, J., *et al.* Unruptured intracranial aneurysms: natural history, clinical outcome, and risks of surgical and endovascular treatment. *Lancet* 2003; **362**: 103–10.

92. Brainin, M., Olsen, T. S., Chamorro, A., *et al.* Organization of stroke care: education, referral, emergency management and imaging, stroke units and rehabilitation. European Stroke Initiative. *Cerebrovasc. Dis.* 2004; **17** (Suppl. 2): 1–14.

93. Hack, W., Kaste, M., Bogousslavsky, J., *et al.* European Stroke Initiative Recommendations for Stroke Management: update 2003. *Cerebrovasc. Dis.* 2003; **16**: 311–37.

94. Schwamm, L. H., Pancioli, A., Acker, J. E., *et al.* Recommendations for the establishment of stroke systems of care: recommendations from the American Stroke Association's Task Force on the Development of Stroke Systems. *Stroke* 2005; **36**: 690–703.

95. Stroke Unit Trialists' Collaboration. Organised inpatient (stroke unit) care for stroke. *Cochrane Database Syst. Rev.* 2002 (1): CD000197.

96. Alberts, M. J., Hademenos, G., Latchaw, R. E., *et al.* Recommendations for the establishment of primary stroke centers. Brain Attack Coalition. *JAMA* 2000; **283**: 3102–9.

97. Duncan, P. W., Zorowitz, R., Bates, B., *et al.*. Management of adult stroke rehabilitation care: a clinical practice guideline. *Stroke* 2005; **36**: e100–43.

98. Tepel, M., van der Giet, M., Schwarzfeld, C., Laufer, U., Liermann, D., & Zidek, W. Prevention of radiographic-contrast-agent-induced reductions in renal function by acetylcysteine. *N. Engl. J. Med.* 2000; **343**: 180–4.

99. Kay, J., Chow, W. H., Chan, T. M., *et al.* Acetylcysteine for prevention of acute deterioration of renal function following elective coronary angiography and intervention: a randomized controlled trial. *JAMA* 2003; **289**: 553–8.

100. Merten, G. J., Burgess, W. P., Gray, L. V., *et al.* Prevention of contrast-induced nephropathy with sodium bicarbonate: a randomized controlled trial. *JAMA* 2004; **291**: 2328–34.

101. Barber, P. A., Demchuk, A. M., Zhang, J., & Buchan, A. M. Validity and reliability of a quantitative computed tomography score in predicting outcome of hyperacute stroke before thrombolytic therapy. ASPECTS Study Group. Alberta Stroke Programme Early CT Score. *Lancet* 2000; **355**: 1670–4.

102. Eastwood, J. D., Engelter, S. T., MacFall, J. F., Delong, D. M., & Provenzale, J. M. Quantitative assessment of the time course of infarct signal intensity on diffusion-weighted images. *AJNR Am. J. Neuroradiol.* 2003; **24**: 680–7.

103. Parizel, P. M., Makkat, S., Van Miert, E., Van Goethem, J. W., van den Hauwe, L., & De Schepper, A. M. Intracranial hemorrhage: principles of CT and MRI interpretation. *Eur. Radiol.* 2001; **11**: 1770–83.

104. Alexandrov, A. V. *Cerebrovascular Ultrasound in Stroke Prevention and Treatment*: Elmsford, NY; Oxford: Blackwell/Futura, 2004.

105. Angeli, S., Del Sette, M., Beelke, M., Anzola, G. P., & Zanette, E. Transcranial Doppler in the diagnosis of cardiac patent foramen ovale. *Neurol. Sci.* 2001; **22**: 353–6.

106. Jauss, M. & Zanette, E. Detection of right-to-left shunt with ultrasound contrast agent and transcranial Doppler sonography. *Cerebrovasc. Dis.* 2000; **10**: 490–6.

107. Toth, C. & Voll, C. Validation of a weight-based nomogram for the use of intravenous heparin in transient ischemic attack or stroke. *Stroke* 2002; **33**: 670–4.

108. Hillbom, M., Erila, T., Sotaniemi, K., Tatlisumak, T., Sarna, S., & Kaste, M. Enoxaparin vs heparin for prevention of deep-vein thrombosis in acute ischaemic stroke: a randomized, double-blind study. *Acta Neurol. Scand.* 2002; **106**: 84–92.

109. Report of the Ad Hoc Committee of the Harvard Medical School to Examine the Definition of Brain Death. A definition of irreversible coma. *JAMA* 1968; **205**: 337–40.

110. Teasdale, G. & Jennett, B. Assessment of coma and impaired consciousness: a practical scale. *Lancet* 1974; **2**: 81–4.

111. Hunt, W. E. & Hess, R. M. Surgical risk as related to time of intervention in the repair of intracranial aneurysms. *J. Neurosurg.* 1968; **28**: 14–20.

112. Teasdale, G. M., Drake, C. G., Hunt, W., *et al.* A universal subarachnoid hemorrhage scale: report of a committee of the World Federation of Neurosurgical Societies. *J. Neurol. Neurosurg. Psychiatry* 1988; **51**: 1457.

113. Rankin, J. Cerebral vascular accidents in patients over the age of 60. *Scott. Med. J.* 1957; **2**: 200–15.

114. Bonita, R. & Beaglehole, R. Modification of Rankin scale: recovery of motor function after stroke. *Stroke* 1988; **19**: 1497–500.

115. Van Swieten, J. C., Koudstaal, P. J., Visser, M. C., Schouten, H. J., & van Gijn, J. Interobserver agreement for the assessment of handicap in stroke patients. *Stroke* 1988; **19**: 604–7.

116. Goldstein, L. B., Bertels, C., & Davis, J. N. Interrater reliability of the NIH stroke scale. *Arch. Neurol.* 1989; **46**: 660–2.

117. Lyden, P., Raman, R., Liu, L., *et al.* NIHSS training and certification using a new digital video disk is reliable. *Stroke* 2005; **36**: 2446–9.